What is being said about
The Ultimate Sports Nutrition Handbook

"This reader friendly book addresses the nutritional concerns of active people and athletes of all ages. If you are a student, coach, athlete, or parent who has an interest in sports nutrition, you must get your hands on *The Ultimate Sports Nutrition Handbook.*"

Jim Clover, A.T.C., M.Ed.
Coordinator of the S.P.O.R.T. Clinic
in Riverside, California

"I would like to express my unlimited admiration to the authors for *The Ultimate Sports Nutrition Handbook.* These women are leaders in the field of sports nutrition. This is a clearly written, easily understood distillation of what an athlete, coach, or even physician should know about nutrition for the athlete. Their clear no nonsense advice for parents dealing with the overweight child or the child who is 'making weight' for wrestling provides clear and easily understood guidelines. The special needs of the athletic woman and a particularly succinct chapter on supplements and nutrition quackery are themselves reason enough to buy this book."

Lyle J. Micheli, M.D.
Director, Division of Sports Nutrition
The Children's Hospital
Boston, Massachusetts

"*The Ultimate Sports Nutrition Handbook* provides a great amount of important and timely information for the coach, athletic trainer, as well as the athlete. Chapters on the child athlete, supplements, and nutrition quackery are excellent descriptions of current concerns for all those involved in finding that 'winning edge'."

Ned Bergert, A.T.,C.
Head Athletic Trainer
California Angels, A.T.,C.

THE
ULTIMATE
SPORTS
NUTRITION
HANDBOOK

Ellen Coleman, RD, MA, MPH
Suzanne Nelson Steen, DSc, RD

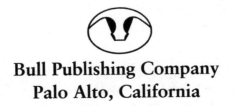

Bull Publishing Company
Palo Alto, California

© 1996 Bull Publishing Company

Bull Publishing Company
P.O. Box 208
Palo Alto, CA 94302-0208
Phone (415) 322-2855 / FAX (415) 327-3300

ISBN 0-923521-34-8

Distributed to the trade by:
Publishers Group West
4065 Hollis Street
Emeryville, CA 94608

Library of Congress Cataloging-in-Publication Data
Coleman, Ellen
    The ultimate sports nutrition handbook / Ellen Coleman,
    Suzanne Nelson Steen.
        p. cm.
    Includes bibliographical references and index.
    ISBN 0-923521-34-8
    1. Athletes—Nutrition—Handbooks, manuals, etc.
    I. Steen, Suzanne Nelson. II. Title.
    TX361-A8C56   1966
    613.2'024796—dc20   96-2593
                                                          CIP

Publisher: James Bull
Production Manager: Helen O'Donnell
Cover Design: Robb Pawlak, Pawlak Design
Interior Design and Composition: Shadow Canyon Graphics

*Dedicated to
David Bull —
an athlete, scholar,
and friend*

CONTENTS

TABLES

FIGURES

1

NUTRIENTS: BUILDING BLOCKS FOR PERFORMANCE

THERE ARE THREE PRIMARY FACTORS that influence your athletic performance: genetics, training, and nutrition. You can't do anything about your heredity, but you do have control over your training and food choices.

Many athletes who train hard to excel are defeated by their diets instead of their competitors. Though a balanced diet won't guarantee you athletic success, an unbalanced diet may undermine your training.

Some athletes will try any dietary regimen in an effort to improve performance, stay healthy, or lose weight. The desire for that elusive "secret ingredient" can cause them to disregard sound nutrition practices and become victims of nutrition fraud. Most popular diets and supplements don't give athletes the results they want, and some dietary fads are actually harmful.

Choosing the proper food is as important to your athletic success as having the most appropriate training program. There are sound dietary strategies that you can use to perform closer to your potential. *The Ultimate Sports Nutrition Handbook* provides the most current information on nutrition for peak athletic performance. It presents sensible nutrition advice that you can put into practice immediately.

NUTRIENTS

Food fulfills three basic needs:

1. It provides energy.
2. It supports new tissue growth and tissue repair.
3. It helps to regulate metabolism.

These three requirements are met by components of foods called nutrients. There are six classes of *nutrients*, and each class has special chemical characteristics suited to meet the specific needs of the body. The six classes are carbohydrates, fats, proteins, vitamins, minerals, and water.

Carbohydrates

Carbohydrates, such as sugar and starch, are the most readily available source of food energy. During digestion and metabolism, all carbohydrates are eventually broken down to the simple sugar glucose for use as the body's principal energy source. Glucose is stored in the muscles and liver as a substance called *glycogen*, which is actually a long chain of glucose molecules hooked together. A high-carbohydrate diet is necessary to maintain muscle glycogen—the primary fuel for most sports. The importance of carbohydrates for peak performance will be discussed in Chapters 2 and 5.

Sugar and starch are grouped together as carbohydrates because they have a chemical similarity. All carbohydrates are made up of one or more simple sugars, the three most common being glucose, fructose, and galactose. The simple sugar glucose connected to fructose forms sucrose, or table sugar. When more than two glucose molecules are connected, they become a starch, or complex carbohydrate. Starches contain anywhere from 300 to 1,000 or more glucose units hooked together.

Though our bodies use both the sugars and the starches for energy, a high-performance diet emphasizes complex carbohydrates. Foods high in complex carbohydrates, such as bread, cereal, rice, beans, pasta, and vegetables, also supply other nutrients, such as vitamins, minerals, protein, and fiber. Sweet foods that are high in sugar (i.e., candy bars, donuts, and cookies) supply carbohydrate, but they also contain a high amount of fat and only insignificant amounts of vitamins and minerals.

Fruit contains the sweetest of all simple sugars—fructose. Because fruit is mostly water, its sugar and calorie content is relatively low. Like starchy foods, most fruits are rich in nutrients and virtually fat free.

Fats

Fats, or lipids, are the most concentrated source of food energy. One gram of fat supplies about nine calories, compared to the four calories per gram supplied by carbohydrate and protein. Fat is the body's only source of a fatty acid called *linoleic acid* that is essential for growth, healthy skin, and hair. Fat insulates and protects the body's organs against trauma and exposure to cold. Fats are also involved in the absorption and transport of the fat-soluble vitamins.

Fats are the source of fatty acids, which are divided into two categories: saturated and unsaturated (including polyunsaturated and monounsaturated fatty acids). These fatty acids differ from each other chemically based on the nature of the bond between carbon and hydrogen atoms.

As a general rule, saturated fat (e.g., butter and lard) is solid at room temperature and is derived mainly from animal sources. Unsaturated fat (e.g., safflower, canola, and corn oil) is liquid at room temperature and is found mainly in plant sources. Palm and coconut oils are exceptions—they are highly saturated vegetable fats. Saturated fat should be restricted because it raises blood cholesterol, which in turn increases the risk of heart disease. The relationship between dietary fat and heart disease will be discussed in Chapters 2 and 7.

Proteins

Protein is a major structural component of all body tissues and is required for tissue growth and repair. Proteins are necessary components of hormones, enzymes, and blood plasma transport systems. Protein is not a significant energy source during rest or exercise. However, the body will use protein for energy if you're not eating enough calories or carbohydrates (i.e., starvation diets and fasting).

The proteins in both animal and plant foods are composed of structural units called *amino acids*. Of the more than 20 amino acids that have been identified, nine must be provided by our diet and are called *essential amino acids*, as shown in Table 1-1. Meat, fish, dairy products, eggs, and poultry contain all nine essential amino acids and are called *complete proteins*. Vegetable proteins, such as beans and grains, are called *incomplete proteins* because they do not supply all the essential amino acids.

The body can make complete proteins if a variety of plant foods—beans, grains, vegetables, fruits, nuts, and seeds—and sufficient calories are eaten during the day. Vegetarians need not worry about combining specific foods within a meal, as the old "complementary protein" theory advised. Well-balanced vegetarian diets may even decrease the risk of heart disease and cancer, because they are lower in fat and higher in complex carbohydrates than the average American diet.

Vitamins

Vitamins are organic molecules (they contain carbon) that the body cannot manufacture but which it requires in small amounts.

TABLE 1-1
Proteins (Essential Amino Acids)

Isoleucine	*Methionine*	*Tryptophan*
Leucine	*Phenylalanine*	*Valine*
Lysine	*Threonine*	*Histidine*

Contrary to what many athletes believe, vitamins do not provide energy. They are metabolic regulators that help govern the processes of energy production, growth, maintenance, and repair. Thirteen vitamins have been identified; each has a specific function in the body and also works in complicated ways with other nutrients. The function and sources of most of the vitamins are shown in Table 1-2.

Vitamins are divided into two groups: water soluble and fat soluble. Fat-soluble vitamins include A, D, E, and K. They are stored in body fat, principally in the liver. Taking a greater amount of vitamins A and D than the body needs over a period of time can produce serious toxic effects. Too much vitamin A can cause loss of appetite, headaches, irritability, liver damage, bone pain, and neurological problems, including brain damage. Too much vitamin D can cause weight loss, vomiting, irritability, and destructive deposits of excess calcium in soft tissues (like the kidneys and lungs), and potentially fatal kidney failure.

While vitamin A is found only in animals, dark orange-yellow and green leafy plants contain substances called *carotenes* (e.g., beta-carotene) that our bodies can convert to vitamin A. Unlike vitamin A, carotene is fairly safe when consumed in large amounts. The body stores excesses of carotenes (which can make the skin look yellow-orange) rather than converting them to vitamin A.

Vitamin C and the B complex vitamins are soluble in water and must be replaced on a regular basis. When you consume more water-soluble vitamins than you need, the excess is eliminated in the urine. Though this increases the vitamin content of

TABLE 1-2
U.S. Recommended Dietary Allowances for Vitamins

ADULT U.S. RDA FEMALE/MALE	FUNCTIONS	SOURCES
Vitamin C 60 mg	Collagen formation, immunity, antioxidant	Citrus fruits, tomatoes, strawberries, potatoes, broccoli, cabbage
Vitamin B$_1$ (Thiamin) 1.1/1.5 mg	Energy production, central nervous system	Meat, whole grain cereals, milk, beans
Niacin 15/19 mg	Energy production, synthesis of fat and amino acids	Peanut butter, whole grain cereals, greens, meat, poultry, fish
Vitamin B$_6$ (Pyridoxine) 1.6/2.0 mg	Protein metabolism, hemoglobin synthesis, energy production	Whole grain cereals, bananas, meat, spinach, cabbage, lima beans
Folacin 180/200 mcg	New cell growth, red blood cell production	Greens, mushrooms, liver
Vitamin B$_{12}$ (Cobalamin) 2 mcg	Energy metabolism, red blood cell production, central nervous system	Animal foods
Vitamin A 800/1,000 mcg	Vision, skin, antioxidant, immunity	Milk, egg yolk, liver, yogurt, carrots, greens
Vitamin D 5 mcg	Formation of bones, aids absorption of calcium	Sunlight, fortified dairy products, eggs, fish
Vitamin E 8/10 mg	Antioxidant, protects unsaturated fats in cells from damage	Vegetable oils, margarines, grains
Vitamin K 65/80 mcg	Blood clotting	Greens, liver

your urine, it doesn't help your performance. Consuming excessive amounts of water-soluble vitamins, such as niacin and B$_6$, can also cause dangerous side effects (see Chapter 8).

Minerals

Minerals are inorganic compounds (they don't contain carbon) that serve a variety of functions in the body. Some minerals, such as calcium and phosphorus, are used to build bones and teeth. Others are important components of hormones, such as iodine in thyroxine. Iron is crucial in the formation of hemoglobin, the oxygen carrier within red blood cells. The function and sources of most of the minerals are shown in Table 1-3.

Minerals also contribute to a number of the body's regulatory functions. These include regulation of muscle contraction, conduction of nerve impulses, clotting of blood, and regulation of normal heart rhythm.

Minerals are classified into two groups based on the body's need. Major minerals, such as calcium, are needed in amounts greater than 100 milligrams per day. Minor minerals or trace elements, such as iron, are required in amounts less than 100 milligrams per day. Calcium and iron are both minerals of concern for athletes, especially women, and are discussed in Chapters 8 and 13.

Water

Water is the most essential of all nutrients for athletes. An adequate supply of water is necessary for control of body temperature (especially during exercise), for energy production, and for elimination of waste products from metabolism.

Dehydration—the loss of body water—impairs athletic performance and increases the risk of heat illnesses (heat exhaustion and heatstroke). Water is probably the nutrient most neglected by athletes.

It's easy to overlook the benefits of water because it is so readily available and inexpensive. The importance of proper fluid replacement for optimum performance will be discussed in Chapter 9.

TABLE 1-3
U.S. Recommended Dietary Allowances for Minerals

ADULT U.S. RDA FEMALE/MALE	FUNCTIONS	SOURCES
Calcium 800 mg	Bone formation, enzyme reactions, muscle contractions	Dairy products, green leafy vegetables, beans
Iron 15/10 mg	Hemoglobin formation, muscle growth and function, energy production	Lean meat, beans, dried fruit, some green leafy vegetables
Magnesium 280/350 mg	Energy production, muscle relaxation, nerve conduction	Grains, nuts, meats, beans
Sodium EMR* 500 mg	Nerve impulses, muscle action, body fluid balance	Table salt, small amounts in most food except fruit
Potassium EMR* 2,000 mg	Fluid balance, muscle action, glycogen and protein synthesis	Bananas, orange juice, fruits, vegetables
Zinc 12/15 mg	Tissue growth and healing, immunity, gonadal development	Meat, shellfish, oysters, grains
Copper ESI* 1.5/3 mg	Hemoglobin formation, energy production, immunity	Whole grains, beans, nuts, dried fruit, shellfish
Selenium 55/70 mcg	Antioxidant, protects against free radicals, enhances vitamin E	Meat, seafood, grains
Chromium ESI* 50/200 mcg	Part of glucose tolerance factor—helps insulin	Whole grains, meat, cheese, beer
Manganese ESI* 2/5 mg	Bone and tissue development, fat synthesis	Nuts, grains, beans, tea, fruits, vegetables
Iodine 150 mg	Regulates metabolism	Iodized salt, seafood
Fluoride 1.5/4 mg	Formation of bones and tooth enamel	Tap water, tea, coffee, rice, spinach, lettuce
Phosphorus 800 mg	Builds bones and teeth, metabolism	Meat, fish, dairy products, carbonated drinks

*EMR—estimated minimum requirement
ESI— estimated safe and adequate dietary intake

NUTRIENTS AND PEAK PERFORMANCE

The key to improved performance and health cannot be found in any one food or supplement, but in a combination of foods that provides the nutrients you need. For peak performance, athletes need to eat a varied diet most of the time. You can't just focus on your pre-exercise meal or what you eat the day before competition.

Though variety is important, don't be overly concerned if you occasionally deviate from a balanced diet. Obtaining a balanced diet isn't as hard as the supplement salespeople would have you believe.

You should be able to get all the nutrients you need by eating a wide variety of foods from the Food Guide Pyramid, which is discussed in the next chapter. Of the 40 known nutrients, 10 are considered *leader nutrients*. If you obtain adequate amounts of leader nutrients from the foods you eat, you probably will obtain the other 30 nutrients as well.

The 10 leader nutrients are protein, carbohydrate, fat, vitamin A, vitamin C, thiamin, riboflavin, niacin, calcium, and iron. The five food groups in the Food Guide Pyramid were developed based on these leader nutrients. The foods in the grain group are high in carbohydrate, thiamin, niacin, and iron. The fruit and vegetable groups contain foods high in vitamins A and C. Meat group foods are high in protein, niacin, iron, and thiamin. Foods in the milk group are good sources of calcium, riboflavin, and protein.

Since no one food or food group supplies all the nutrients you need, it's important to choose a wide variety of foods from the five groups in the Pyramid. By eating at least the minimum number of servings from each food group daily, you can be reasonably assured you're getting the nutrients you need for optimum performance. The next chapter will discuss how to develop a training meal plan to get the most out of your workouts.

2

TRAINING DIETS FOR PERFORMANCE AND HEALTH

EVENTUALLY ALMOST ALL ATHLETES will encounter problems due to haphazard or irregular eating habits. Nutrition-related difficulties are usually due to inadequate carbohydrate intake and may result in reduced speed, impaired endurance, and difficulty concentrating. Unwanted weight loss or weight gain may also be the result of poor food choices. Sound eating habits can help to prevent these problems and promote optimal performance. A healthy diet should also help to prevent major health problems—heart disease, stroke, and cancer.

There is no single diet for athletes, since each sport makes nutritional demands that require individual attention for peak performance (see Chapter 4). However, the nutritional guidelines developed to promote health establish a good foundation for athletes who desire peak performance. This chapter discusses these guidelines and how they make up a training diet for athletes and other active people. The nutritional requirements for specific sports are addressed in later chapters.

FOOD GUIDE PYRAMID

The *Food Guide Pyramid* (Figure 2-1) shows the foods that should be included in a healthful diet and in what amounts. The grain group forms the base of the pyramid, the fruit and vegetable groups are on the second tier, and the meat and dairy groups are on the third tier. Because fats and sweets should be consumed in limited amounts, these items are grouped in a small

FIGURE 2-1
The Food Guide Pyramid

KEY
• Fat (naturally occurring and added)   ▼ Sugars (added)
These symbols show that fat and added sugars come mostly from fats, oils, and sweets, but can be part of or added to foods from the other food groups as well.

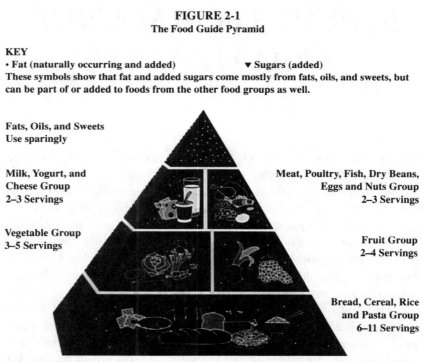

Fats, Oils, and Sweets
Use sparingly

Milk, Yogurt, and
Cheese Group
2–3 Servings

Meat, Poultry, Fish, Dry Beans,
Eggs and Nuts Group
2–3 Servings

Vegetable Group
3–5 Servings

Fruit Group
2–4 Servings

Bread, Cereal, Rice
and Pasta Group
6–11 Servings

The Food Guide Pyramid is a guide to daily food choices from the five food groups. Each food group provides some, but not all, of the nutrients you need.

■ **Source:** U.S. Department of Agriculture and U.S. Department of Health and Human Services.

TABLE 2-1
What Counts as 1 Serving?

BREAD, CEREAL, RICE AND PASTA GROUP
1 slice bread
½ cup cooked rice or pasta
½ cup cooked cereal
1 oz ready-to-eat cereal

VEGETABLE GROUP
½ cup chopped raw or cooked vegetables
1 cup leafy raw vegetables
½ cup tomato or vegetable juice

FRUIT GROUP
1 piece fruit or melon wedge
¾ cup juice
½ cup canned fruit
¼ cup dried fruit

MILK, YOGURT AND CHEESE GROUP
1 cup milk or yogurt
1½ oz natural cheese
2 oz processed cheese

MEAT, POULTRY, FISH, DRY BEANS, EGGS AND NUTS GROUP
2½–3 oz cooked lean meat, poultry, or fish
½ cup cooked beans, or 1 egg, or 2 tbsp. peanut butter as 1 oz lean meat

FATS, OILS AND SWEETS
Use sparingly *especially if you need to lose weight.*

The amount you eat may be more than one serving. For example, a dinner portion of spaghetti would count as 2 or 3 servings.

---

section at the top of the pyramid. Alcoholic beverages are also part of this group. Fats, sweets, and alcohol are often called "empty calories" because they are high in calories but low in most nutrients.

Americans, and particularly athletes, should eat heartily from the grain, vegetable, and fruit groups because these groups have the highest recommended number of servings and are nutrient-

TABLE 2-2
How Many Servings Do You Need Each Day?

CALORIE LEVEL*	WOMEN AND SOME OLDER ADULTS	CHILDREN, TEEN GIRLS, ACTIVE WOMEN, MOST MEN	TEEN BOYS AND ACTIVE MEN
	About 1,600	**About 2,200**	**About 2,800**
Bread Group	6	9	11
Vegetable Group	3	4	5
Fruit Group	2	3	4
Milk Group	2–3**	2–3**	2–3**
Meat Group	2	2	3
	for a total of 5 ounces	*for a total of 6 ounces*	*for a total of 7 ounces*

*These are the calorie levels if you choose low-fat, lean foods from the 5 major food groups and use foods from the fats, oils, and sweets group sparingly.
**Women who are pregnant or breast-feeding, teenagers, and young adults to age 24 need 3 servings.
■ **Source:** U.S. Department of Agriculture and the U.S. Department of Health and Human Services.

rich sources of carbohydrate. Table 2-1 indicates what counts as a serving from each group.

The number of calories the Food Guide Pyramid provides will vary, depending on the selection of foods within the groups and the number of servings eaten (see Table 2-2). The minimum number of servings from the Food Guide Pyramid provides about 1,600 calories if you choose low-fat, lean foods from the five groups and use items from the fats and sweets group sparingly. Eating the minimum number of servings from the pyramid will promote body fat loss for most athletes while providing adequate nutrients. High-calorie items such as fats, sweets, and alcohol should be limited when body fat reduction is desired. Effective strategies for body fat loss will be discussed in Chapter 11.

Consuming the maximum number of servings (with a limited use of fats and sweets) provides about 2,800 calories. Athletes who have higher caloric needs for weight maintenance or weight gain can eat a greater number of servings from the food groups by eating between-meal snacks. Emphasis should be placed on the grain, fruit, and vegetable groups because they generally provide more carbohydrate and less fat than the meat and milk groups. There's also no harm in eating a reasonable amount of sweets to supply needed calories once you've met your nutrient needs. Effective strategies for weight gain will be discussed in Chapter 12.

DIETARY GUIDELINES FOR AMERICANS

In 1980 a joint committee of the U.S. Department of Agriculture and the U.S. Department of Health and Human Services issued the first set of Dietary Guidelines for Americans. These guidelines, designed to reduce the risk of chronic disease, were revised most recently in 1995 to reflect current scientific knowledge on diet and health. The Food Guide Pyramid is based on these recommendations. Here are the guidelines:

Eat a variety of foods. Unlike many popular diets, good nutrition is based more on common sense than on glitzy schemes. Different foods, rather than a single food or supplements, are necessary to supply the nutrients essential to good health and performance. The essential nutrients that your body must obtain on a daily basis include water, carbohydrates, protein, essential fatty acids, vitamins, and minerals. The Guidelines recommend a specific number of servings per day from the grain, fruit, vegetable, milk, and meat groups to meet these requirements, which are illustrated by the Food Guide Pyramid (see Figure 2-1, page 12).

Balance the food you eat with physical activity. Maintain or improve your weight. Individuals who are overweight or obese are at greater risk for many medical disorders than are those who are near or at desirable body weight. Among overweight individuals, a 10–15% weight loss is reasonable and maintainable. This amount reduces some of the health complications associated with excess weight and eliminates the need to diet down to "ideal" body weight. Instead of a short-lived fad diet, permanent lifestyle changes are required that include increased physical activity and decreased consumption of calories.

The Guidelines also take into account the waist–hip ratio, since excess fat in the abdomen (rather than the hips or thighs) increases the risk of heart disease and diabetes. The Guidelines recommend that women not exceed a waist–hip ratio of 0.8 and that men not exceed 1.0. For a person losing excess weight, the Guidelines recommend a gradual loss of 0.5 to 1.0 pound per week, based on the size of the person. The rationale is that the slower the weight is taken off, the more likely it is to stay off. Optimal weight (based on body composition) for athletes and other active people is discussed in Chapter 10.

Choose a diet with plenty of grain products, vegetables, and fruits. High-carbohydrate foods are generally rich in vitamins, minerals, and fiber, and they are low in fat. Foods rich in fiber can reduce the risk of constipation, certain colon disorders, and possibly even colon cancer.

Choose a diet low in fat, saturated fat, and cholesterol. The average American consumes an average of 37% of total calories as fat. Excess dietary and body fat has been associated with the development of heart disease, obesity, diabetes, and cancer. Total fat should be limited to 30% of total calories and saturated fat limited to 10% of calories. If you consume 2,000 calories a day, your maximum fat intake should be 600 calories (30% × 2,000). This corresponds to 66 grams of fat (600 divided by 9, the number of calories in a gram of fat). As shown by the sample food label in Figure 2-2, one serving of the food has 3 grams of fat.

It's also important to restrict cholesterol intake to less than 300 milligrams per day. Cholesterol is found only in animal products and is generally found in foods high in saturated fat. However, foods that are high in saturated fat are not necessarily high in cholesterol. Watching your saturated fat intake is more important than watching your cholesterol intake to maintain healthy levels of cholesterol in your blood.

Choose a diet moderate in sugars. Sugar and sugar-rich sweets are high in calories and low in nutrients. Sugars can also contribute to tooth decay.

FIGURE 2-2
A Sample Food Label

Reading the label tells more about the food and what you are getting. What you see on the food label—the nutrition and ingredient information—is required by the government. This shows what the new label looks like and explains some of its new features.

NUTRITION FACTS TITLE
The new title "Nutrition Facts" signals the new label.

NEW LABEL INFORMATION
The new nutrient list covers those most important to your health. You may have seen this information on some old labels, but it is now required.

VITAMINS AND MINERALS
Only two vitamins, A and C, and two minerals, calcium and iron, are required on the food label. A food company can voluntarily list other vitamins and minerals in the food.

LABEL NUMBERS
Numbers on the nutrition label may be rounded for labeling.

SERVING SIZE
Similar food products now have similar serving sizes. This makes it easier to compare foods. Serving sizes are based on amounts people actually eat.

% DAILY VALUE
shows how a food fits into a 2,000 calorie reference diet. You can use % Daily Value to compare foods and see how the amount of a nutrient in a serving of food fills in a 2,000 calorie reference diet.

DAILY VALUES FOOTNOTE
Daily Values are the new label reference numbers. These numbers are set by the government and are based on current nutrition recommendations.

Some labels list the daily values for a daily diet of 2,000 and 2,500 calories. Your own nutrient needs may be less than or more than the Daily Values on the label.

Nutrition Facts

Serving Size 1 cup (228g)
Servings Per Container 2

Amount Per Serving

Calories 90   Calories from Fat 30

% Daily Value*

Total Fat 3g	5%
Saturated Fat 0g	0%
Cholesterol 0 mg	0%
Sodium 300 mg	13%
Total Carbohydrate 13g	4%
Dietary Fiber 3g	12%
Sugars 3g	

Protein 3g

Vitamin A 80%	•	Vitamin C 60%
Calcium 4%	•	Iron 4%

*Percent Daily Values are based on a 2,000 calorie diet. Your daily values may be higher or lower depending on your calorie needs:

		Calories	2,000	2,500
Total Fat	Less than		65g	80g
Sat Fat	Less than		20g	25g
Cholesterol	Less than		300mg	300mg
Sodium	Less than		2,400mg	2,400mg
Total Carbohydrate			300g	375g
Dietary Fiber			265g	30g

Calories per gram:

Fat 9   •   Carbohydrate 4   •   Protein 4

Choose a diet moderate in salt and sodium. The American diet is incredibly high in sodium, which is consumed mainly as salt. By weight, 40% of salt is sodium (the other 60% is chloride). The average American consumes 17 times more salt than the body needs—salt that is added to processed foods and at the table. The sodium in the body acts like a sponge, causing the body to retain water and in some cases to raise blood pressure. Reducing sodium in the diet (Table 2-3) will benefit people whose blood pressure rises with excessive sodium in their diets. The body requires only 1,100 to 1,300 milligrams of sodium per day. While the Dietary Guidelines for Americans don't give a specific limitation for sodium intake, the National Academy of Sciences recommends no more than 2,400 milligrams a day—the amount in a teaspoon of table salt. The sodium needs of active people will be discussed in Chapter 9.

If you drink alcoholic beverages, do so in moderation. Because alcohol is practically devoid of nutrients (but not calories), when incorporated into the diet it often replaces more nutritious foods. Alcohol consumption is associated with several medical problems and contributes prominently to four of the ten leading causes of death in the United States (cirrhosis of the liver, motor vehicle and other accidents, suicide, and homicides).

Any alcohol consumed affects the structure and function of the cells in the liver and the brain. Chronic consumption can lead to liver disease as well as an increased risk for oral, esophageal, and other cancers. Two drinks at any given time in the day and a total of 14 drinks per week represent the upper limit of moderate alcohol intake; anything above this is defined as a problem with alcohol. One drink is considered to be 12 ounces of beer, 5 ounces of wine, or 1½ ounces of 80 proof liquor.

DEVELOPING A HIGH-CARBOHYDRATE DIET

If you want to be sure you're eating enough carbohydrate, you can keep track of the number of grams you're eating each day. Depending on the intensity and duration of your sport or activity,

---

TABLE 2-3
Tips for Reducing Salt Intake

- Reduce or omit table salt added to meals and used in cooking.

- Reduce obviously salty foods such as salted crackers, chips, cheese curls, pretzels, popcorn, salted nuts, olives, pickles, sauerkraut, pickled herring, anchovies.

- Reduce smoked and cured meats and fish such as ham, bacon, sausage, hot dogs, corned beef, bologna, salami, pepperoni, pastrami, lox, processed cheeses.

- Use smaller amounts of seasonings and condiments such as ketchup, steak sauce, mustard, relish, soy sauce, MSG (monosodium glutamate), Worcestershire sauce, garlic salt. Experiment with other spices such as curry, dill, thyme, pepper, lemon, onion, garlic, or chives.

- Check labels of commercially prepared foods such as canned or frozen meals, dried mixes, bouillon cubes (unless labeled as "low sodium" or "sodium free") to determine sodium content.

---

you should be consuming 6 to 10 grams of carbohydrate per kilogram of body weight. We'll discuss carbohydrate needs of specific sports and activities in Chapters 4 and 5.

A practical high-carbohydrate diet can be created by using the *food exchange system*. The exchange lists are the basis of a meal-planning system developed by the American Dietetic Association and the American Diabetes Association.

There are six food-planning exchange lists: grain, vegetables, fruit, meat, milk, and fat (Table 2-4). Each lists foods that have about the same number of carbohydrate, protein, fat, and calories. Any food on a list can be exchanged, or traded, for any other food on the same list.

These food exchange lists can be used to plan diets from 1,500 to 4,000 calories a day (see Table 2-5). These diets supply about 60% carbohydrate, 15% protein, and less than 25% fat. Because the grain, fruit, and vegetable exchanges are high in carbohydrate and low in fat, they are emphasized. Foods from the milk list are also good sources of carbohydrate. To keep your

TABLE 2-4
Food Group Exchanges

STARCH/BREAD/GRAINS
(80 CALORIES)

15 grams carbohydrate
3 grams protein
0 grams fat

½ cup pasta, barley, cooked cereal
⅓ cup rice or dried cooked peas/beans
½ cup corn, peas, winter squash
1 small (3 oz) baked potato
4–6 crackers
1 slice bread or 6 inch tortilla
½ bagel, English muffin, pita
¼ cup dry flaked cereal
3 cups popcorn, no oil or butter
¾ oz pretzels

MEAT AND MEAT ALTERNATIVES
(55–100 CALORIES)

0 grams carbohydrate
7 grams protein
3–8 grams fat

1 oz poultry, fish, beef, pork, lamb, etc.
¼ cup tuna, salmon, cottage cheese
2 tbsp. peanut butter
1 egg
1 oz cheese
tofu (2½ inch × 2¾ inch × 1 inch)

VEGETABLES
(25 CALORIES)

5 grams carbohydrate
2 grams protein
0 grams fat

½ cup cooked vegetables
1 cup raw vegetables
½ cup tomato or vegetable juice

MILK
(90–150 CALORIES)

12 grams carbohydrate
8 grams protein
0–5 grams fat

1 cup milk: nonfat, low-fat, 1%, whole
1 cup yogurt: nonfat, low-fat, 1%, whole

FRUIT
(60 CALORIES)

15 grams carbohydrate
0 grams protein
0 grams fat

1 medium fresh fruit
1 cup berries or melon
½ cup canned fruit (without sugar)
½ cup fruit juice
¼ cup dried fruit

FAT
(45 CALORIES)

0 grams carbohydrate
0 grams protein
5 grams fat

1 tsp. margarine, oil, butter, mayonnaise
2 tsp. diet margarine, diet mayonnaise
1 tbsp. salad dressing, cream cheese,
* cream, nuts*
2 tbsp. diet salad dressing, sour cream
1 slice bacon

TABLE 2-5
Training Diet Meal Plans

FOOD GROUP	NUMBER OF EXCHANGES PER CALORIE LEVEL					
	1,500	**2,000**	**2,500**	**3,000**	**3,500**	**4,000**
Milk	3	3	4	4	4	4
Meat	5	5	5	5	6	6
Fruit	5	6	7	9	10	12
Vegetable	3	3	3	5	6	7
Grain	7	11	16	18	20	24
Fat	2	3	5	6	8	10

intake of fat low, choose low-fat or nonfat foods from the milk and meat lists.

Sugary foods such as cookies, cake, pie, soft drinks, and candy can supply additional carbohydrate but are low in most other nutrients. Though there's no harm in eating some high-carbohydrate "empty calories" once you've met your nutrient needs, you can't go wrong adding extra servings of complex carbohydrates and fruit.

NUTRITION COUNSELING

Beware of self-proclaimed nutrition "experts" who promote questionable foods, supplements, and fad diets. The title "nutritionist" can be used by anyone, regardless of training. Under the heading "nutritionist," you have more than a 50% chance of finding a person with phony credentials or someone who delivers false information. If you want individual nutrition counseling, consult a registered dietitian (credentials abbreviated R.D.).

A registered dietitian is a health-care professional who is educated in nutrition and food science. For a person to become an R.D., the American Dietetic Association (ADA) requires specific course work from an accredited university (minimum of a bachelor of science degree), completion of a nutrition internship at an approved hospital, and the passing of a national certification exam. Registered dietitians are required to continue their professional education by attending scientific meetings or by writing scientific papers and giving lectures to colleagues.

You can find an R.D. by requesting a referral from your physician or by contacting the nutrition department of a hospital, clinic, or community health agency. You can also check in the phone book under dietitians, nutritionists, and weight control—remember to look for the R.D. after the name.

There are registered dietitians who specialize in sports nutrition. They usually belong to the Sports, Cardiovascular, and Wellness Nutrition Group (abbreviated SCAN) of the ADA. You can be referred to SCAN members in your geographic area by calling the American Dietetic Association at 1-800-366-1655.

3

THE ENERGY DEMANDS OF EXERCISE

YOUR BODY MUST BE CONTINUOUSLY SUPPLIED with energy to perform its many complex functions. As the body's energy demands increase with exercise, there must be a way to provide this additional energy or you would stop moving.

This chapter describes the body's energy systems and how food provides energy for exercise. It also discusses the factors that determine the type of fuel your muscles use during exercise. After learning about exercise fuel usage, you'll have a better appreciation of the importance of carbohydrate in your diet.

ATP—THE ENERGY CURRENCY

The energy-rich chemical compound *adenosine triphosphate,* or simply *ATP,* is used for all energy-requiring processes within the cell (Figure 3-1, page 25). The energy released from the breakdown of ATP is used to power all body functions, such as muscle contraction, so ATP is considered the "energy currency" of the cell. Another energy-rich compound called *creatine phosphate,* or *CP,* provides a small reserve of quick energy (Figure 3-2, page 25). The energy released from the breakdown of ATP and CP stores sustains all-out exercise (such as sprinting 100 meters) for about 6 to 8 seconds.

ATP must be continuously produced to provide a steady supply of energy. The muscle cells produce and maintain ongoing stores of ATP, utilizing glucose from carbohydrates, fatty acids from fats, and to a small extent, amino acids from proteins. The body extracts the energy from dietary or body stores of carbohydrate, fat, and protein to rebuild the energy-rich ATP.

ENERGY PRODUCTION

Chains of chemical reactions use food, oxygen, and water to supply energy at rest and during exercise. This is referred to as *metabolism*. ATP is produced continuously within muscle cells through two important related energy systems. The *anaerobic* or *lactic-acid* energy system doesn't require oxygen and provides immediate energy. It soon needs help, however, from the *aerobic* energy system, which depends on a steady supply of oxygen.

For a limited period of time, about a minute, you can rely on the anaerobic system. The anaerobic system supplies most of the energy for an all-out 440-yard sprint. It allows you to briefly exercise at a level that exceeds your ability to provide oxygen to your muscles. Anaerobic metabolism is a built-in survival mechanism—it protects us when we have a sudden need to fight or flee from danger.

When you exercise beyond several minutes, such as running a mile, your body needs a continuous supply of oxygen. The aerobic energy system provides almost all of your energy during exercise that lasts four minutes or longer.

ANAEROBIC PATHWAY

Glucose is the only fuel that can be used when oxygen is not available. Glucose is stored in the muscles and liver as glycogen—

FIGURE 3-1
Adenosine Triphosphate (ATP)

Adenosine triphosphate (ATP) is the immediate source of energy for muscle contraction. When the end phosphate is split off, energy is released.

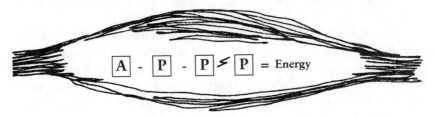

FIGURE 3-2
Creatine Phosphate (CP)

This energy-rich compound splits to release energy for the rapid resynthesis of ATP.

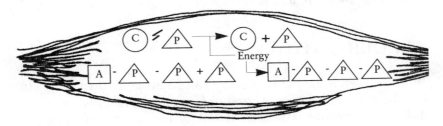

FIGURE 3-3
The Lactic Acid Energy System

In the lactic acid energy system, muscle glycogen (carbohydrate) can break down to form ATP in the absence of adequate oxygen, but lactic acid is formed.

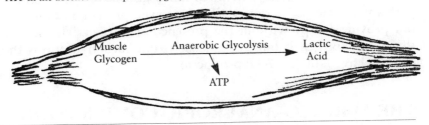

which is actually a long chain of glucose molecules hooked together. In the anaerobic pathway, glucose is broken down to a substance called *pyruvate*. When oxygen is not available, pyruvate is converted into lactic acid, forming two molecules of ATP, as shown in Figure 3-3 (page 25).

Although the anaerobic pathway provides energy rapidly, there is a limit to the amount of lactic acid the body can tolerate. This is why anaerobic metabolism can fuel exercise for only a short period of time. When oxygen becomes available, lactic acid is converted back into pyruvate or burned directly by the muscles for energy. Lactic acid can also go to the liver and be converted back into glucose.

The anaerobic pathway provides you with energy for all-out effort lasting up to 60 seconds, such as long sprints. It also provides energy for bursts that are common in sports such as soccer, basketball, football, and tennis.

AEROBIC PATHWAY

When oxygen is available, glucose can be broken down more efficiently, without being converted to lactic acid. As shown in Figure 3-4, when glucose is broken down in the aerobic pathway, 36 ATP molecules are produced. This is 18 times more energy than when glucose is converted to lactic acid in the anaerobic pathway.

Fatty acids (from fat in the diet and body) and amino acids (the building blocks of protein) can also go through the aerobic pathway to release energy as ATP. However, protein and fat cannot provide energy without the presence of oxygen. This means that when oxygen is limited, glucose (from carbohydrate) is the only fuel available for ATP production.

THE AEROBIC–ANAEROBIC COMBINATION

At the beginning of exercise it takes time for the heart and blood vessels to get oxygen-rich blood to the muscles. During this lag

FIGURE 3-4
The Anaerobic and Aerobic Reaction Systems Working Together

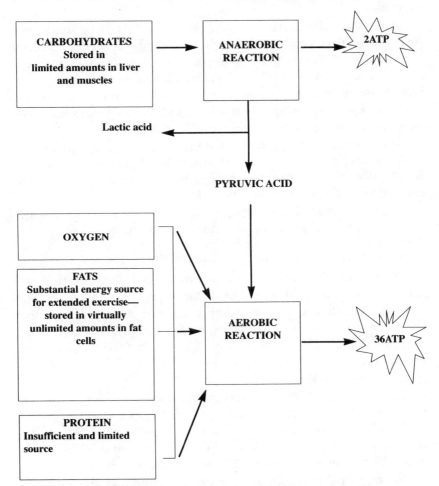

When enough oxygen is present in the muscle, the more efficient aerobic reaction system operates to provide the energy (ATP) used for muscle contraction. The aerobic system is very efficient and can produce up to 18 times the amount of ATP produced by the anaerobic system.

The aerobic system can utilize fats and, to a lesser extent, proteins, which are stored in virtually unlimited amounts in the body.

time, anaerobic ATP production supplies most of the energy for exercise.

After several minutes, oxygen becomes available and aerobic ATP production provides most of the energy needed to sustain exercise. However, when the exercise becomes too intense for enough energy to be produced aerobically (as when running up a hill or sprinting in a marathon), the body relies on the anaerobic pathway for more energy. This additional ATP is generated at the cost of increasing the lactic acid level in the blood.

In an event lasting several minutes, such as a half-mile run, the contributions of aerobic and anaerobic ATP are about equal. As the distance (or time) increases, the contribution of aerobically produced energy increases.

Although anaerobic energy production determines performance during sprint-type activities, the capacity to produce ATP aerobically determines endurance performance. Thus, the availability of oxygen in large part determines the potential for aerobic exercise.

Your capacity for exercise intensity and for duration are inversely related. That is, as the distance (or time) increases, you have to reduce your intensity, or pace. For example, a runner can't run a marathon (26.2 miles) as fast as a 10-kilometer race (6.2 miles). You can perform only at a certain percentage of your maximum aerobic capacity (abbreviated as VO_{2max}) for any given distance or time.

The aerobic pathway cannot tolerate the same level of intensity as the duration increases. A trained runner can run a mile at 100% of her aerobic capacity. In a 5-kilometer race (3.1 miles), she can use about 95% of her aerobic capacity. In a 10-kilometer race, she can average about 90% of her aerobic capacity.

During prolonged endurance exercise, there is an additional reason why you cannot perform close to your aerobic capacity for the entire distance. During endurance exercise that exceeds 90 to 120 minutes, your muscle glycogen stores become progressively lowered. When this happens, you must either stop exercising or continue at a much slower pace. Muscle glycogen depletion is a well-recognized limitation to endurance performance and will be discussed further in Chapter 5.

DETERMINANTS OF EXERCISE FUEL USAGE

A variety of factors determine which type of fuel your muscles will use during exercise. These include exercise intensity, exercise duration, and your training level.

Intensity

The intensity of exercise is particularly important in determining your muscles' energy source. High-intensity, short-duration exercise (such as sprinting) relies on the anaerobic pathway for energy production. Only glucose, derived primarily from the breakdown of muscle glycogen, can be used as fuel.

When glucose is broken down anaerobically, muscle glycogen is used 18 times faster than when glucose is broken down aerobically. A more rapid rate of muscle glycogen breakdown will also occur during high-intensity exercise (e.g., over 70% of your aerobic capacity) when the anaerobic pathway is pulled in to assist the aerobic pathway in ATP production. Extended mixed anaerobic–aerobic intermittent exercise like football drills, soccer, basketball, and running or swimming intervals also causes a greater breakdown of muscle glycogen. Figure 3-5 shows energy systems for competitions of varying duration.

What about aerobic exercise such as distance running? Muscle glycogen and blood glucose supply half of the energy for aerobic exercise during a moderate workout (at or below 60% of aerobic capacity) and supply nearly all the energy during a hard workout (above 80% of aerobic capacity).

Exercise of low to moderate intensity (up to 60% of aerobic capacity) can be fueled almost entirely aerobically. The hormonal changes that occur with exercise—increased epinephrine (adrenaline) and decreased insulin levels—prompt your fat (adipose) tissue to release fatty acids into the bloodstream. These fatty acids, combined with fat pools within the muscle, supply about half of the energy for low- to moderate-intensity exercise at or below 60% of aerobic capacity. Muscle glycogen and blood glucose supply the rest.

FIGURE 3-5
Energy Systems for Competitions of Varying Duration

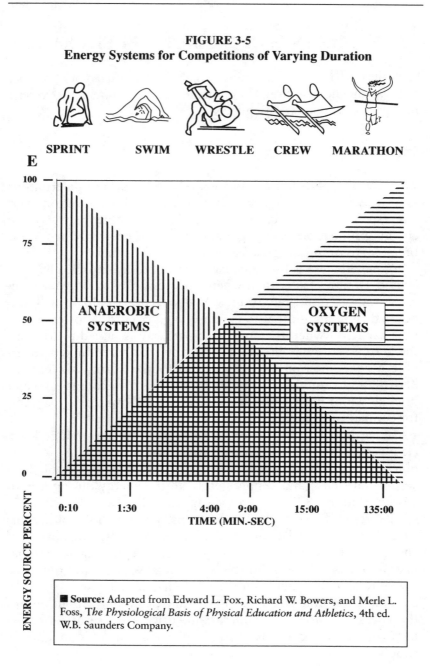

SPRINT   SWIM   WRESTLE   CREW   MARATHON

ANAEROBIC SYSTEMS

OXYGEN SYSTEMS

E

ENERGY SOURCE PERCENT

100 —

75 —

50 —

25 —

0 —

0:10   1:30   4:00   9:00   15:00   135:00

TIME (MIN.-SEC)

■ **Source:** Adapted from Edward L. Fox, Richard W. Bowers, and Merle L. Foss, *The Physiological Basis of Physical Education and Athletics*, 4th ed. W.B. Saunders Company.

There are several reasons that fat cannot be used as fuel during high-intensity exercise (above 70% of aerobic capacity). First, the breakdown of fat to ATP is a slow process and cannot supply ATP fast enough to provide energy for high-intensity exercise.

Also, glucose provides more calories per liter of oxygen than does fat. Glucose delivers 5.10 calories per liter of oxygen, and fat delivers 4.62 calories per liter of oxygen. When less oxygen becomes available, as during high-intensity exercise, it is a distinct advantage for the muscles to use glucose because less oxygen is needed to produce energy.

Last, the shift in fuel from fat to glycogen as the exercise intensity increases is also partly due to the accumulation of lactic acid. During high-intensity exercise, lactic acid hinders the use of fat by the muscles. Thus, the muscles must rely more on glycogen for energy production.

Duration

The duration of exercise also defines whether the fuel used will be muscle glycogen or fat. The longer you exercise, the greater the contribution of fat as fuel. Fat can supply as much as 60–70% of the energy needs for moderate-intensity exercise lasting 4 to 6 hours.

As the duration of exercise increases, the intensity must decrease, since there is a limited supply of stored glycogen. When muscle glycogen stores are low, fat breakdown supplies most of the energy needed for exercise. However, fat can be used as fuel only up to 60% of aerobic capacity. Also, a certain level of carbohydrate breakdown is necessary for fats to be burned for energy.

As a result of the relationship between exercise intensity and duration, muscle glycogen is the predominant fuel for most types of exercise. It takes at least 20 minutes for fat to be available to the muscles as fuel in the form of free fatty acids. Most people don't train long enough to burn significant amounts of fat as fuel during the exercise session itself. Also, most people train and compete at an exercise intensity of 70% of aerobic capacity or above, which decreases the use of fat as fuel.

This does not mean that you have to work out for a long time to lose body fat. When your workout creates a caloric deficit, the body will pull from its fat stores at a later time to make up that caloric deficit. We'll discuss the benefits of exercise for body fat loss in Chapters 7 and 11.

Because fat is an important fuel source during prolonged exercise, some endurance athletes think they should eat a high-fat diet. This isn't necessary, since even the leanest athletes have more fat stored than they will ever use during exercise. The goal is to increase the utilization of fat as fuel through endurance training. Also, as Chapter 7 points out, a high-fat diet can increase your risk of health problems.

Keep in mind that eating too much fat also decreases your carbohydrate intake. As Chapter 5 indicates, a low-carbohydrate diet lowers muscle glycogen stores. This decreases your ability to sustain high-intensity exercise and limits your endurance. Thus, the ideal diet supplies enough carbohydrate (60–70% carbohydrate, or 6 to 10 grams per kilogram of body weight) to ensure optimal muscle glycogen stores.

Training Level

Your aerobic capacity ($\dot{V}O_{2max}$) will also determine what fuel your muscles use during exercise. The delivery of blood by the heart and the extraction of oxygen from the blood by the muscles determine your aerobic capacity. Endurance training increases both the maximum delivery of blood by the heart and the extraction of oxygen from the blood by the muscles.

Thus, endurance training increases your ability to perform more aerobically at the same absolute level of exercise. In terms of fuel usage, endurance training enables you to use more fat and less glycogen at the same absolute level of exercise, compared to less fit people. Your ultimate aerobic capacity seems to be genetically determined, but whether or not you reach your full potential depends on training.

Untrained people start to accumulate lactic acid in their blood at about 50% of their aerobic capacity. Trained people start to accumulate lactic acid in their blood at about 70% of aerobic capacity. The point at which lactic acid accumulates is called the *blood lactate threshold*.

When lactic acid begins to accumulate at 70% of an individual's aerobic capacity, the person's blood lactate threshold is said to be 70% of VO_{2max}. Remember that lactic acid speeds up the rate of muscle glycogen breakdown by interfering with the use of fat as fuel. A higher blood lactate threshold is one reason that trained people use more fat and less glycogen at the same absolute level of exercise.

Endurance training also increases the ability of the aerobic energy system in your muscles to use fat for energy. When more fat is burned, less glycogen is used. This "glycogen sparing" effect of fat utilization is beneficial during prolonged exercise since muscle glycogen depletion limits performance. Using more fat and less glycogen aids endurance because muscle glycogen stores are limited and fat stores are abundant.

Lastly, endurance training increases the capacity of the muscles to store glycogen. Thus, endurance training confers a dual performance advantage: The muscle glycogen stores are higher at the onset of exercise, and the person uses them up at a slower rate.

4

NUTRITIONAL REQUIREMENTS FOR DIFFERENT SPORTS

MANY ATHLETES ARE CONFUSED about what to eat before they train and compete. This chapter provides recommendations for your pre-exercise meal and discusses how the duration of your sport or activity influences your nutritional requirements.

Keep in mind that eating well during training is just as important as eating well before or during competition. Proper dietary habits help you to train harder so that you're better prepared for competition.

EATING BEFORE EXERCISE

Many athletes train and compete in the morning without eating. This overnight fast lowers liver glycogen stores—the body's main source of blood glucose. When liver glycogen stores become depleted, blood sugar drops and you can feel fatigued and light-headed. Eating a high-carbohydrate meal before morning exercise will help to maintain blood glucose levels so that you can perform at your best.

During exercise, athletes rely primarily on their pre-existing muscle glycogen and fat stores. Although the pre-exercise meal doesn't contribute immediate energy for exercise, it can provide energy when the athlete exercises longer than an hour. The carbohydrate in the meal elevates blood glucose to provide energy for the working muscles. The pre-exercise meal also helps prevent feelings of hunger and weakness, which can harm performance.

Try to consume your carbohydrate-rich meal one to four hours before training or competition. This allows adequate time for food to empty from the stomach. Exercising with a full stomach can cause indigestion, nausea, and vomiting as blood is diverted from the stomach to the muscles.

The amount to consume depends on the timing of the meal. To avoid potential gastrointestinal distress, the size of the meal should be reduced the closer to exercise it is consumed. For example, a small meal of 300 to 400 calories is appropriate an hour before exercise, whereas a large meal of 700 to 800 calories can be consumed four hours before exercise.

Good examples of high-carbohydrate foods for breakfast meals include bread products (adding jam or jelly increases the carbohydrate content), fruit, nonfat or low-fat yogurt, sports bars, and liquid meals. Fruit juices and nonfat or 1% fat milk are good high-carbohydrate beverages. You can also use high-carbohydrate liquid supplements, which we'll discuss in the next chapter. Table 4-1 provides examples of pre-event meals. These meals contain plenty of carbohydrates and limit the amount of fat and protein.

Fatty foods should be limited because they delay stomach emptying and can contribute to a sluggish, heavy feeling. Many high-protein foods (e.g., eggs and cheese) are also high in fat and should be limited. In contrast, carbohydrates are rapidly digested to provide a readily available source of energy.

High-fiber foods (especially those high in bran) should be limited as they may cause abdominal cramping and necessitate a bathroom break during exercise. While this is merely annoying during training, it can be disastrous during competition. It's also a good idea to minimize gas-forming foods such as beans, broccoli,

---

TABLE 4-1
Examples of Pre-event Meals

BREAKFAST

Orange juice
Blueberry pancakes with syrup
Bagel
Low-fat yogurt
Banana

Cranberry juice
Cornflakes
Low-fat milk
Apple muffin

....

LUNCH/DINNER

Chicken sandwich on whole-wheat roll
Fruit cup
Fig bar
Frozen low-fat yogurt

Low-fat milk
Pasta with tomato sauce
Salad with tomato, carrots, cucumbers, and mushrooms
Italian bread
Fresh fruit
Low-fat milk
Sherbet

Baked potato with low-fat cheese
Cornmeal muffin
Low-fat vanilla milk shake

Thick crust cheese and mushroom pizza
Low-fat milk
Fresh fruit
Bread sticks

✔ **Note:** Caloric intake depends on length of time before event.

cauliflower, and onion. Extremely salty foods can cause fluid retention and a bloated feeling.

Experimenting with a variety of pre-event meals in training helps to determine what foods are most likely to settle well during competition. Many athletes are tense before competition, which slows down the digestive process. This means that even familiar, well-tolerated foods may take longer to digest. Never try an untested food or fluid before competition, especially a major event. The result may be severe indigestion, impaired performance, or an allergic reaction.

Drinking fluids with your pre-exercise meal and right before exercise helps to ensure that you're properly hydrated. Caffeine-containing beverages such as coffee, tea, and soda may cause problems for some athletes, particularly children. The side effects of consuming caffeine—agitation, nausea, muscle tremors, palpitations, and headache—can impair performance.

Keep in mind that caffeine is also a diuretic. Excessive caffeine intake can stimulate the production of urine and cause water losses. This may contribute to dehydration and reduced endurance in hot weather if the athlete doesn't hydrate properly. We'll discuss hydration guidelines and appropriate fluid-replacement beverages in Chapter 9.

Some athletes have "lucky" foods they associate with winning. As long as these foods don't harm the athlete's performance, it's fine to include them even if they don't meet the recommendations for pre-event meals.

Liquid Meals

A number of commercially formulated liquid meals are available, as shown in Table 4-2. Their fluid and carbohydrate content makes them a desirable meal choice either before competition or during day-long competitions such as swim meets, track meets, and tennis, volleyball, and wrestling.

Liquid meals have several advantages over conventional meals. They leave the stomach more rapidly than regular meals

TABLE 4-2
Nutrition Beverages

BEVERAGE	FLAVORS	CALORIES (per 8-oz serving)	CARBOHYDRATE (grams)	PROTEIN (grams)	FAT (grams)
GatorPro® Sports Nutrition Supplement The Gatorade Company	Chocolate, vanilla	360	58	16	7
Sport Shake® Mid-America Farms	Chocolate, vanilla, strawberry	310	45	11	10
Endura Optimizer® Unipro, Inc.	Chocolate, vanilla, orange	260	57	11	less than 1
Sego Very® Pet, Inc.	Chocolate, chocolate malt, strawberry, vanilla	180	27–34	9	1–4
Protein Repair Formula® PurePower Sports Nutrition	Vanilla	200	26	20	1.5
Metabolol II® Champion Nutrition	Plain	260	40	20	2

and thus help to avoid pre-competition nausea. Liquid meals also produce a low stool residue and so help to keep immediate weight gain to a minimum. Because of their low residue, liquid meals are also less likely to cause a bathroom break during exercise. They also satisfy hunger and supply energy without giving an uncomfortable feeling of fullness. Many athletes value a feeling of "lightness," especially as they enter major competition.

Homemade liquid meals can be concocted by mixing 1% fat milk, fruit, and nonfat dry milk powder in a blender. For added variety, you can add cereal, yogurt, and flavoring (vanilla and chocolate). Sugar and honey may also be used for additional sweetness and carbohydrate. There are also several brands of "instant breakfast" powders that can be mixed with milk.

EATING FOR SHORT-DURATION EVENTS

There are two important steps to get ready for an all-out event lasting up to four minutes. First, the muscle stores of ATP, CP, and glycogen should not be exhausted by hard exercise immediately before the event. Also, the athlete's caloric intake should be adequate for several days prior to the event. Athletes should eat at least the minimum number of servings from the Food Guide Pyramid during training.

During track and swim meets, athletes are often involved in several events. Though each event may not last long, the repeated bursts of all-out effort may significantly reduce muscle glycogen stores. Ideally, enough time should be allowed between events to restore muscle glycogen to optimal levels.

Recovery periods are also necessary to clear the muscles of the build-up of lactic acid from anaerobic metabolism. Glycogen depletion from repetitive events and the accumulation of lactic acid can both impair performance.

Athletes in short-term events require water and carbohydrate throughout the day of the meet. Some athletes may be reluctant to eat and drink since they have to compete again. However, failing to do so can cause a deterioration in performance, particularly toward the end of the day. Because everything you eat before an event may be considered a pre-event meal, it's important to consider the amount of time the athlete has between competitions.

If there is less than an hour between competitions, you can drink water, sports drinks, and diluted fruit juices. When there are several hours between events, you can eat easily digestible carbohydrate-rich foods such as fruit, grain products (e.g., fig bars, bagels, graham crackers), low-fat yogurt, sports bars, and liquid meals. When the events are separated by three hours or more, high-carbohydrate meals may be eaten.

EATING FOR INTERMEDIATE-LENGTH EVENTS

A variety of sports require intense exertion for periods of 4 to 10 minutes and longer. The mile run, wrestling matches, middle-distance swimming events, and rowing contests all demand maximal effort without rest. Muscle glycogen is the predominant fuel for these events. Although aerobic metabolism supplies most of the athlete's energy needs, the intense nature of such exercise precludes the use of fat as fuel.

Athletes in these events must ensure that their muscle glycogen stores are adequate when they enter competition. The events themselves usually aren't long enough to cause muscle glycogen depletion. However, heavy training in preparation for competition can significantly lower muscle glycogen stores. If muscle glycogen has not been replenished prior to competition (restoration of glycogen stores takes 24 to 48 hours), the athlete's performance will suffer. To guarantee optimal muscle glycogen stores prior to competition, the athlete should taper training and eat a high-carbohydrate diet.

Athletes in intermediate events must also be well hydrated before competition to perform at their best. Some athletes do not adequately replace fluid losses between training sessions and so enter competition in a dehydrated state. This impairs performance and increases the risk of heat illnesses.

EATING FOR ENDURANCE EVENTS

Athletes involved in distance running, cross-country skiing, triathlons, and distance cycling often train heavily and compete in events that significantly lower their muscle and liver glycogen stores. Muscle glycogen depletion is a well-recognized limitation to endurance exercise that exceeds 90 to 120 minutes. Athletes who train exhaustively on successive days must consume adequate carbohydrate to prevent cumulative depletion of muscle glycogen.

Endurance athletes should consume a carbohydrate-rich meal one to four hours before prolonged training and competition to help provide glucose for the muscles to use when they're running low on glycogen. Carbohydrate feeding during events lasting several hours or longer also improves endurance.

Endurance athletes who compete for longer than 90 minutes can improve their performance by maximizing their muscle glycogen stores during the week prior to the event. This dietary program, called carbohydrate loading, will be discussed in the next chapter.

Proper hydration is the most important nutritional concern during prolonged endurance exercise. An endurance athlete can collapse from heat exhaustion or heatstroke long before muscle glycogen stores are depleted. Endurance athletes in particular are susceptible to impaired performance from chronic dehydration. This will be addressed further in Chapter 9.

5

CARBOHYDRATES: YOUR HIGH-OCTANE FUEL

MUSCLE GLYCOGEN IS THE PREFERRED FUEL for most types of exercise. Replenishing and maintaining glycogen stores during training and prior to competition requires a carbohydrate-rich diet. This chapter reviews carbohydrate requirements for training and the role of complex carbohydrates and sugar in your diet. Carbohydrate loading, carbohydrate intake during endurance exercise, and carbohydrate needs for recovery are also discussed.

CARBOHYDRATE NEEDS FOR TRAINING

Muscle glycogen depletion can occur over repeated days of heavy training when muscle glycogen breakdown exceeds its replacement. When this happens, the glycogen stores drop lower with each successive day, and you can't maintain your usual training intensity.

It's common to be tired after several days of high-intensity workouts, especially if you train for several hours a day. However,

43

training glycogen depletion (and/or dehydration) should be suspected when you're always tired and unable to maintain your usual training intensity. The deterioration in performance and feeling of sluggishness associated with training glycogen depletion is often referred to as "staleness" and blamed on overtraining.

Training glycogen depletion can occur while training for sports that require repeated, near-maximal bursts of effort (such as soccer, basketball, and football) as well as during endurance exercise. A sudden weight loss of several pounds (due to glycogen and water loss) often accompanies training glycogen depletion. Athletes who don't consume enough carbohydrate or calories and/or don't take rest days are prime candidates.

Training glycogen depletion can be prevented by a carbohydrate-rich diet and periodic rest days to give the muscles time to rebuild their stores. Carbohydrate is essential for glycogen synthesis and should provide at least 60% of the athlete's calories, or about 6 grams of carbohydrate per kilogram of body weight.

The typical American diet of 46% carbohydrate (about 4 to 5 grams of carbohydrate per kilogram) doesn't supply enough carbohydrate to enable you to recover adequately from hard workouts lasting an hour.

The recommendations for carbohydrate are given in grams per kilogram (gm per kg) because this is an easy way to determine how much you need. One kilogram equals 2.2 pounds. For example, a 154-pound (70-kg) person who trains strenuously for an hour needs 420 gm of carbohydrate daily. Table 5-1 gives some examples of high-carbohydrate foods. You can determine the carbohydrate content of different foods by reading food labels.

The food exchange lists (see Chapter 2) can be used to develop a high-carbohydrate diet. As a general guide, starchy foods and fruits provide the highest amount of carbohydrate (15 gm) per serving. A serving of starch consists of one slice of bread or small tortilla, ½ cup pasta or cooked cereal, ⅓ cup cooked rice or beans, or 1 small potato. A serving of fruit is one medium-size fruit, 1 cup berries or melon, ½ cup juice, or ¼ dried fruit. Milk is the next highest source, providing 12 gm of carbohydrate for 1 cup of milk or yogurt (choose nonfat or 1% fat products to keep your fat intake down). Vegetables provide 5 gm of carbohydrate per ½ cup cooked vegetables, 1 cup raw vegetables, or ½ cup tomato or vegetable juice.

A diet containing 8–10 gm of carbohydrate per kg is recommended when you're training hard for several hours or more daily. As we'll discuss later in this chapter, a high-carbohydrate diet is even more critical for recovery from prolonged, heavy exercise.

THE ROLE OF SUGAR AND SUGAR MYTHS

Sugary foods such as cakes, cookies, pies, soft drinks, and candy can be helpful for increasing carbohydrate and calorie intake during training. However, these foods should be eaten in addition to, not in place of, complex carbohydrate foods. Otherwise, when sugar replaces complex carbohydrates in the athlete's diet, the intake of vitamins, minerals, and fiber will be reduced. Remember that sugar can also contribute to tooth decay. Many sugary baked goods and candy are also high in fat.

Despite popular press claims, brown sugar, date sugar, honey, and molasses are not nutritionally superior to table sugar. Though they do contain trace amounts of some vitamins and minerals, consuming these so-called natural sugars will not add significant nutritional value to your diet.

Some endurance athletes take fructose, thinking that is it superior to glucose or other sugars. Fructose causes a lower insulin response than glucose, which has led some athletes to think that it is a better energy source.

However, consuming fructose does not improve endurance and has even been shown to harm performance. You store twice as much muscle glycogen after eating glucose or sucrose compared to eating fructose. Also, fructose is far more likely to cause gastrointestinal distress, even in small amounts. For this reason, glucose, maltodextrins (glucose polymers), and sucrose are the major carbohydrate sources in sports drinks. Maltodextrins are created by breaking down cornstarch into small glucose chains (polymers).

TABLE 5–1
High-Carbohydrate Foods

FOOD GROUP	CALORIES	CARBOHYDRATES (GRAMS)
Milk		12
Low-fat (2%) milk (1 cup)	*121*	*12*
Skim milk (1 cup)	*86*	*26*
Chocolate milk (1 cup)	*208*	*30*
Pudding, any flavor (½ cup)	*161*	*34*
Frozen yogurt, low-fat (1 cup)	*220*	*42*
Fruit-flavored low-fat yogurt (1 cup)	*225*	
Beans		22
Blackeye peas (½ cup)	*134*	*44*
Pinto beans (1 cup)	*235*	*48*
Navy beans (1 cup)	*259*	*26*
Refried beans (½ cup)	*142*	*45*
Garbanzo beans (chickpeas) (1 cup)	*269*	*45*
White beans (1 cup)	*249*	
Fruits and Vegetables		
Fruits		
Apple (1 medium)	*81*	*21*
Apple juice (1 cup)	*111*	*28*
Applesauce (1 cup)	*232*	*60*
Banana (1)	*105*	*27*
Canteloupe (1 cup)	*57*	*14*
Dates, dried (10)	*228*	*61*
Fruit Roll-Ups (1 roll)	*50*	*12*
Grapes (1 cup)	*114*	*28*
Grape juice (1 cup)	*96*	*23*
Orange (1)	*65*	*16*
Orange juice (1)	*112*	*26*
Pear (1)	*98*	*25*
Pineapple (1 cup)	*77*	*19*
Prunes, dried (10)	*201*	*53*
Raisins (2/3 cup)	*302*	*79*
Raspberries (1 cup)	*61*	*14*
Strawberries (1 cup)	*45*	*11*
Watermelon (1 cup)	*50*	*12*
Vegetables		20
Three-bean salad (½ cup)	*90*	*8*
Carrots (1 medium)	*31*	*21*
Corn (½ cup)	*89*	*45*
Lima beans	*217*	*12*
	63	*50*

TABLE 5-1
High-Carbohydrate Foods (continued)

FOOD GROUP	CALORIES	CARBOHYDRATES (GRAMS)
Peas, green (½ cup)	63	12
Potato (1 large)	220	50
Sweet Potato (1 large)	118	28
Grain		
Bagel (1)	165	31
Biscuit (1)	103	13
White bread (1 slice)	61	12
Whole-wheat bread (1 slice)	55	11
Breadsticks (2 sticks)	77	15
Cornbread (1 square)	178	28
Cereal, ready-to-eat (1 cup)	110	24
Oatmeal (½ cup)	66	12
Cream of Rice (¼ cup)	95	21
Cream of Wheat (¾ cup	96	20
Flavored oatmeal, Quaker instant (1 packet)	110	25
Graham crackers (2 squares)	60	11
Saltines (5 crackers)	60	10
Triscuit crackers (3 crackers)	60	10
Pancake (4-inch diameter)	61	9
Waffles (2, 3.5″×5.5″)	130	17
Rice (1 cup)	223	50
Rice, brown (1 cup)	232	50
Hamburger bun (1)	119	21
Hotdog bun (1)	119	21
Noodles, spaghetti (1 cup)	159	34
Flour tortilla (1)	85	15
Oatmeal raisin cookie	62	9
Pizza (cheese, 1 slice)	290	39
Popcorn, plain (1 cup, popped)	26	6
English muffin	154	130
Fig bar (1)	50	10
Granola bar (low-fat, 1)	109	16
Pretzels (1 oz)	106	21

Consuming sugar before anaerobic exercise such as sprinting or weight lifting will not improve performance, because the body relies on stored ATP and muscle glycogen for these tasks. It won't provide you with a sudden burst of energy, allowing you to exercise harder or longer. To the contrary, eating too much sugar immediately before or during exercise can increase the risk of gastrointestinal problems in the form of cramps, nausea, diarrhea, and bloating.

THE ROLE OF COMPLEX CARBOHYDRATES AND FRUITS

As we discussed in Chapter 2, your primary food sources should be the grain products, vegetables, and fruits found at the bottom of the Food Guide Pyramid. These foods promote good health and athletic performance. Grain products, vegetables, and fruits supply vitamins, minerals, and fiber along with their carbohydrate.

The dietary fiber found in whole grains, vegetables, and fruit smay reduce your risk of heart disease and certain cancers. The American Dietetic Association recommends consuming 20–35 gm of dietary fiber daily, but the average American takes in only 10–15 gm daily. The soluble fiber found in beans, fruits, oats, and vegetables can help to lower the cholesterol level in your blood. Because high blood cholesterol is a major risk factor for heart disease (see Chapter 7), consuming more soluble fiber may help reduce your risk for heart disease.

Insoluble fiber found in whole-grain products and bran speeds up the movement of food through the gastrointestinal tract. Insoluble fiber may reduce your risk for colon cancer and other bowel disorders. (Fruits and vegetables high in beta-carotene and vitamin C may also help to prevent some kinds of cancer.) Insoluble fiber also provides a feeling of satiety, which is important for weight control, and can reduce constipation. Table 5-2 lists the fiber content of selected foods.

Grain products, fruits, and vegetables are "nutrient dense" — they supply a significant amount of nutrients for their calories. Let's compare a small baked potato with a third of a candy bar, which both contain about 100 calories. The potato provides ample vitamin C, with a small amount of protein, B vitamins, about a half-dozen minerals, and fiber. The third of the candy bar provides the same amount of energy, about three times as much fat, and little or no fiber, vitamins, and minerals.

Contrary to popular belief, starches such as bread, cereal, potatoes, corn, beans, rice, and pasta contribute significantly fewer calories for a given amount than foods with a high fat or sugar content. The "diet lunch" of a hamburger patty and a scoop of cottage cheese provides a lot of fat calories.

By replacing fats and sugary foods in the diet, complex carbohydrates actually facilitate weight loss because they contain fewer calories. Also, the naturally occurring sugars in fruit make them ideal for a sweet, low-calorie treat.

COMMERCIAL CARBOHYDRATE SUPPLEMENTS

Some athletes train so heavily that they have difficulty eating enough food to meet their carbohydrate needs. This can happen for several reasons.

Often, the stress of hard training can decrease appetite, resulting in reduced consumption of calories and carbohydrate. Eating a large volume of food can also cause gastrointestinal discomfort and interfere with training. And some athletes spend so much time training that there aren't many rest hours available for replenishment.

Athletes who have problems consuming carbohydrate can use a commercial high-carbohydrate supplement. Table 5-3 compares selected high-carbohydrate beverages. These products should not replace regular food but are designed to supply additional calories and carbohydrate when needed. If the athlete can consume an adequate amount of food, these products are unnecessary.

TABLE 5–2
Fiber Content of Foods

	Serving Size	Grams of Dietary Fiber
BREADS		
Bran muffin	1 medium	3
Whole-wheat bread	1 slice	2
White, pumpernickel or rye	1 slice	1
CEREALS AND PASTA		
Kellogg's All-Bran	1 ounce	9
Whole-wheat pasta	1 cup	5
Kellogg's Bran Flakes	1 ounce	4
General Mills Cheerios	1 ounce	2
Post Grape-Nuts	1 ounce	2
Oatmeal	1 cup	2
Popcorn	1 ounce	2
General Mills Wheaties		
Pasta	1 cup	1
Kellogg's Corn Flakes	1 ounce	1
Cooked brown or white rice	½ cup	1
FRUITS AND NUTS		
Almonds	¼ cup	5
Dried Prunes	3	4
Apple (with skin)	1 medium	3
Banana	1 medium	3
Dried dates	5	3
Nectarine	1 medium	3
Peach (with skin)	1 medium	3
Roasted peanuts	¼ cup	3
Strawberries	1 cup	3
Cantaloupe	¼ cup	2
Orange	1 medium	2
Smooth peanut butter	2 tbsp.	2
Walnut pieces	¼ cup	2
Grapefruit	½	1
COOKED LEGUMES		
Kidney beans	½ cup	9
Baked beans	½ cup	7
Navy beans	½ cup	5
Pinto beans	½ cup	5
Lentils	½ cup	2

TABLE 5-2
Fiber Content of Foods (continued)

	Serving Size	Grams of Dietary Fiber
VEGETABLES		
Cooked frozen peas	½ cup	4
Baked potato (with skin)	1 medium	4
Cooked broccoli tops	½ cup	3
Cooked young carrots	½ cup	3
Cooked corn	½ cup	3
Cooked green beans	½ cup	2
Brussels sprouts	½ cup	2
Cooked sweet potato	½ cup	2
Raw lettuce	½ cup	1
Sliced raw mushrooms	½ cup	1
Fresh tomato	½ medium	1

High-carbohydrate supplements should be taken before or after exercise, either with meals or between meals. They are too concentrated in carbohydrate to be used as fluid-replacement drinks during exercise.

CARBOHYDRATE LOADING

During endurance exercise that exceeds 90 to 120 minutes, such as marathon running, muscle glycogen stores become progressively lower. When they drop to critically low levels (the point of glycogen depletion), high-intensity exercise cannot be maintained. In practical terms, the athlete is exhausted and must drastically reduce the pace.

Athletes using muscle glycogen supercompensation techniques, or carbohydrate loading, can increase their muscle glycogen stores by 50–100%. The greater the pre-exercise muscle glycogen content, the greater the endurance potential. Table 5-4 gives an overview of the diet and training regimen used for carbohydrate loading.

TABLE 5–3
High-Carbohydrate Beverages

Beverage	Flavors	Carbohydrate Ingredient	Carbohydrate % (concentration) 12-oz Serving	Carbohydrate	Sodium
GatorLode® High Carbohydrate Loading and Recovery Drink The Gatorade Company	Lemon, citrus, banana	Malrodextrin, glucose	20	70	95
Carboplex® Unipro, Inc.	Plain	Maltrodextrin	24	82	0
Carbo Power® Nature's Best Food Supplements	Lemonade, strawberry, fruit punch, orange, grape, tea	Maltodextrin, high-fructose corn syrup	18	64	76
Ultra Fuel® Twin Labs	Lemon, lime, grape, fruit punch, orange	Maltodextrin, glucose, fructose	21	75	0
ProOptibol® 105 Next Nutrtion	Wild berry	Glucose fructose	19	66	
Cybergenics Cybercharge® L & S Research Corp.	Lemon, lime, grape	Glucose, polymers, fructose	21	75	15
Carbo Fire ® Weider Health & Fitness	Tropical punch, orange	Glucose, polymers fructose	24	83	60

TABLE 5–4
Training and Diet Regimen for Glycogen Loading

	TRAINING	EATING	
DAY 1	*90 min • 70-75% $\dot{V}O_{2max}$*	*50% Carbohydrate*	*5gm/kg*
DAY 2	*40 min • 70–75% $\dot{V}O_{2max}$*	*50% Carbohydrate*	*5gm/kg*
DAY 3	*40 min • 70–75% $\dot{V}O_{2max}$*	*50% Carbohydrate*	*5gm/kg*
DAY 4	*20 min • 70–75% $\dot{V}O_{2max}$*	*70% Carbohydrate*	*10gm/kg*
DAY 5	*20 min • 70–75% $\dot{V}O_{2max}$*	*70% Carbohydrate*	*10gm/kg*
DAY 6	*Rest*	*70% Carbohydrate*	*10gm/kg*
DAY 7	*EVENT*	*EVENT*	

Six days before competition, you exercise moderately hard (70% of aerobic capacity) for 90 minutes to lower muscle glycogen stores. On that day and the next two days, you consume a normal diet providing about 50% carbohydrate (5 gm/kg). On the second and third days, training is decreased to 40 minutes at aerobic capacity. On the next two days, you eat a high-carbohydrate diet providing about 70% carbohydrate (10 gm/kg) and reduce training to 20 minutes at 70% of aerobic capacity. On the day before competition, you rest but maintain the high-carbohydrate diet.

Endurance training is the primary stimulus for muscle glycogen synthesis. This means the athlete must be endurance trained or carbohydrate loading won't work. Also, the exercise to lower glycogen stores must be the same as the athlete's competitive event because glycogen stores are specific to the muscle groups used. For example, a runner needs to decrease her or his stores by running rather than cycling.

It's essential that you reduce training for the three days prior to the event. Too much exercise during this period will use too much of the stored glycogen and defeat the purpose of the whole process. The final three days, when you rest and eat a high-carbohydrate diet, is the real "loading" phase of the regimen.

If you have difficulty consuming enough carbohydrate from food, a high-carbohydrate commercial supplement can be added to intake. Athletes who have diabetes or high blood triglyceride levels may have problems if they carbohydrate-load. They should check with their doctor before attempting the regimen.

For each gram of glycogen stored, additional water is stored. Some athletes note a feeling of stiffness or heaviness associated with the increased glycogen storage. These sensations will dissipate with exercise.

Carbohydrate loading will help only athletes engaged in continuous endurance exercise lasting longer than 90 minutes. Greater than normal muscle glycogen stores won't enable the athlete to exercise harder during shorter duration exercise such as a 10-kilometer run. In fact, the stiffness and heaviness associated with the increased glycogen stores can hurt performance during shorter events.

The increased muscle glycogen stores enable the athlete to maintain high-intensity exercise longer but will not affect the pace for the first hour of exercise. The athlete won't be able to go out faster, but will be able to maintain the same pace longer.

CARBOHYDRATE FEEDINGS DURING ENDURANCE EXERCISE

Carbohydrate feedings during endurance exercise lasting longer than an hour and a half may improve endurance by providing glucose for the muscles to use when their glycogen stores have dropped to low levels.

The liver supplies glucose to maintain blood sugar for proper functioning of the central nervous system. As the muscles run out of glycogen, they will begin to take up some of the blood glucose, placing a drain on the liver glycogen stores. The longer the exercise session, the greater the utilization of blood glucose by the muscles for energy.

When the liver glycogen is depleted, the blood glucose drops. Though a few athletes experience symptoms of low blood sugar (hypoglycemia) such as dizziness, most athletes are forced to reduce their exercise intensity due to muscular fatigue.

The improved performance associated with carbohydrate feedings during prolonged exercise is due to the maintenance of blood glucose levels. The dietary carbohydrate supplies glucose for the muscles at a time when their glycogen levels are diminished. Thus, the production of ATP from carbohydrate continues at a high rate and performance is enhanced. Remember that ATP (energy) production is faster from carbohydrate than from fat.

Endurance athletes should take in 30 to 60 grams of carbohydrate (120 to 240 calories) every hour. This amount can be obtained from either carbohydrate-rich foods (fruits, grain products, liquid meals, and sports bars) or sports drinks. Sports drinks are a practical source of carbohydrate since they replace fluid losses as well.

Drinking 4–8 oz of a sports drink containing 5–8% carbohydrate (e.g., Gatorade and Exceed) every 15 minutes supplies carbohydrate and also aids in hydration. Eating one banana, four graham crackers, 4 oz of a liquid meal (e.g., GatorPro, Sustacal) or half of a sports bar (e.g., Power Bar, Gatorbar) every hour also provides the recommended amount of carbohydrate.

Athletes should eat before they feel tired or hungry, usually within 30 minutes into exercise. Consuming small amounts at frequent intervals (every 30 to 60 minutes) will help prevent gastrointestinal upset. The athlete's foods and fluids should be easily digestible, familiar (tested in training), and enjoyable (to encourage eating and drinking).

CARBOHYDRATE NEEDS FOR RECOVERY FROM EXERCISE

The replacement of muscle glycogen stores following strenuous training is important to minimize chronic fatigue. Based on the time spent training, athletes should consume 6–10 gm of carbohydrate per kg daily (about 60–70% calories from carbohydrate).

It's also important to consume carbohydrate immediately (within 30 minutes) after heavy exercise lasting several hours. Taking in high-carbohydrate fluids and foods right after prolonged training and competitions increases muscle glycogen storage and may improve your recovery time. Replenishing muscle glycogen stores after exercise is particularly beneficial for athletes who train hard several times a day. This will enable them to get the most out of their second workout.

Many athletes aren't hungry after heavy training. If this is the case, they can consume a high-carbohydrate drink such as fruit juice or a commercial high-carbohydrate supplement. This will also promote rehydration.

Athletes exercising hard for several hours a day should consume 1.5 gm of carbohydrate per kg within 30 minutes of exercise, followed by an additional 1.5 gm/kg feeding 2 hours later. The first carbohydrate feeding could be a high-carbohydrate beverage and the second feeding could be a high-carbohydrate meal.

6

PROTEIN: THE GREAT DEBATE

MANY BODY BUILDERS AND STRENGTH ATHLETES (weight lifters, football players, and athletes in some field events) believe that they require increased amounts of protein to perform at their best. They are encouraged by "pumping iron" magazines and locker-room talk to consume high-protein diets and take protein/amino acid supplements. These athletes are frequently told that additional protein will increase their muscle mass, thereby improving their potential for strength development.

Endurance athletes have also been encouraged by advertisements in popular athletic magazines to consume specific amino acids during exercise to improve endurance and again following exercise to enhance their recovery.

This chapter addresses the protein needs of strength and endurance athletes. The protein content of foods, protein supplements, and amino acid supplements are also discussed.

EXERCISE AND PROTEIN

Athletes do need more protein than sedentary people. Exercise may promote a loss of muscle protein through reduced protein synthesis and increased protein breakdown. The hormonal changes that occur during exercise—increased epinephrine (adrenaline) and decreased insulin levels—may be responsible for these effects of exercise on protein metabolism.

Exercise may also promote body protein loss in other ways. Protein has been found in the urine of athletes after marathon runs and after football, basketball, and handball games. Protein may also be lost through sweating.

Regular physical training tends to reduce muscle protein breakdown and protein loss from the body. Although some protein breakdown may occur during exercise, protein build-up is enhanced in the recovery period that follows. Regular exercise seems to increase the effectiveness of the protein synthesis that occurs during recovery.

PROTEIN AS FUEL

As discussed in Chapter 2, several factors influence what the muscles use for fuel during exercise. The most important of these factors are the duration of exercise and the carbohydrate content of the diet.

When muscle glycogen stores are low, due to prolonged exercise or a low-carbohydrate diet, protein may contribute as much as 10% of the energy needed for exercise. However, when muscle glycogen stores are high, the contribution of protein for energy is no more than about 5%. Athletes will also use more protein for fuel when they don't eat enough calories. Consuming a high-carbohydrate diet during repeated days of heavy training helps to maintain muscle glycogen stores and reduces the use of protein as fuel.

PROTEIN NEEDS OF ATHLETES

The recommended dietary allowance (RDA) for protein for sedentary adults is 0.8 gm per kg of body weight per day. Athletes need 50–100% more protein than the adult RDA. Endurance athletes need 1.2 gm per kg daily and may benefit from 1.4 gm per kg during prolonged endurance exercise. Strength athletes need 1.2 gm per kg daily and may benefit from 1.7 gm per kg during periods of muscle building.

An increased protein intake appears to be more important during the early stages of training than later in the training program. Strength athletes initially require more protein to support increases in their muscle mass—the existing muscle fibers become larger. Endurance athletes initially need more protein to support increases in the aerobic enzymes (proteins) in the muscle, red blood cell formation, and the formation of myoglobin (an oxygen carrier in the muscle similar to hemoglobin).

Athletes can obtain 1.2–1.7 gm of protein per kg when their diet provides 12-15% of calories as protein. This amount of protein is consistent with the dietary recommendations for athletes: 60–70% carbohydrate, 12–15% protein, and 20–30% fat.

The growing athlete needs more protein relative to body weight than does the adult athlete to support growth requirements. A diet supplying 15% of the calories as protein, or 1.2–1.7 gm per kg daily, should meet the needs of most children and adolescents in sports.

These protein guidelines assume that the athlete is consuming enough calories. Total caloric intake is more important than increased protein intake when trying to increase muscle mass. (This is discussed further in Chapter 12.) Many athletes mistakenly emphasize protein intake over caloric intake when trying to "bulk up." Athletes who have difficulty gaining weight generally aren't eating enough calories.

Athletes need more protein when they don't eat enough calories due to heavy training or when they reduce their caloric intake to keep weight low for a sport such as wrestling, gymnastics, figure skating, or ballet. The athlete's protein requirement increases because the protein is used for energy rather than for muscle growth and repair. When athletes eat enough to fulfill their caloric requirement, they usually take in more than enough protein.

PROTEIN IN FOOD

Athletes can easily obtain enough protein through their diet. The average sedentary American consumes about 100 gm of protein per day for a total protein intake of about 1.4 gm per kg, or 16% of total calories. About 70% of this protein comes from animal sources, which, as discussed in Chapter 1, contain all the essential amino acids.

Athletes consume more protein when their caloric intake increases as a result of training. For example, a 70 kg athlete who gradually increases his caloric intake from 2,500 to 3,500 calories during training would increase his protein intake from 94 gm per day to 131 gm per day if 15% of his calories came from protein. His daily protein intake relative to body weight would increase from 1.3 gm/kg to 1.8 gm/kg, which would be more than adequate.

Good sources of complete proteins are meat, poultry, fish, dairy products, and eggs. An ounce of meat, poultry, or cheese or one egg each supplies about 7 gm of protein containing all the essential amino acids. Milk and yogurt are also excellent complete protein sources, with 8 oz supplying 8 gm of protein. To reduce dietary fat, athletes should emphasize lean meat, chicken or turkey without the skin, and nonfat or 1% fat dairy products. A list of the protein content in some foods in provided in Table 6-1.

A well-balanced vegetarian diet can easily supply enough protein, as long as the protein sources are varied and the athlete eats enough calories. Guidelines for vegetarians are supplied in Table 6-2 (page 62). Whole grains, beans, seeds, nuts, and vegetables supply adequate amounts of essential and nonessential amino acids.

AMINO ACID SUPPLEMENTS

Amino acid supplements are popular among athletes such as body builders and weight lifters who are trying to "bulk up." Proponents of amino acid supplements claim that certain amino acids increase muscle mass and decrease body fat.

TABLE 6-1
Protein Content in Some Common Foods

FOOD	AMOUNT	PROTEIN (GRAMS)
Milk List		
Milk, whole	1 cup	8
Milk, skim	1 cup	8
Cheese, cheddar	1 oz	7
Yogurt	1 cup	8
Meat List		
Beef, lean	1 oz	8
Chicken, breast	1 oz	8
Luncheon meat	1 oz	5
Fish	1 oz	7
Eggs	1	6
Navy beans, cooked	½ cup	7
Peanuts, roasted	½ cup	18
Peanut butter	1 tbsp.	4
Starch/Bread List		
Macaroni and cheese	½ cup	9
Peas, green	½ cup	4

✔ **Note:** Protein (grams) may vary slightly from the food exchange lists since these data were derived from food analyses reported by the United States Department of Agriculture.

Arginine and ornithine are particular favorites since they supposedly stimulate the secretion of growth hormone, thereby increasing muscle mass and decreasing body fat. Consuming large amounts of these amino acids may cause a temporary rise in growth hormone levels, but there is no proof that this increases muscle mass or reduces body fat. Weight lifting and endurance training both significantly increase growth hormone levels. Combining the supplements with exercise does not increase growth hormone levels above those seen with exercise.

Athletes may hear that only a small amount of the amino acids in foods is digested and absorbed. This is not correct. The truth is that about 95–99% of the amino acids from animal sources and about 90% of the amino acids from vegetable sources are digested and utilized by the body.

TABLE 6-2
Daily Food Guide for Vegetarians

FOOD GROUP: BREAD, CEREALS, RICE, PASTA
Recommended servings: 6 or more
Serving Sizes: *1 slice bread, ½ bagel or English muffin, ½ cup cooked cereal,*
rice, or pasta, 1 oz dry cereal

FOOD GROUP: VEGETABLE
Recommended serving: 4 or more
Serving Sizes: *½ cup cooked , 1 cup raw*

FOOD GROUP: BEANS AND OTHER MEAT SUBSTITUTES
Recommended servings: 2 to 3
Serving Sizes: *½ cup cooked beans, 4 oz tofu, 8 oz soy milk, 2 tbsp.*
nuts or seeds (used sparingly if on a low-fat diet)

FOOD GROUP: FRUIT
Recommended servings: 3 or more
Serving Sizes: *1 piece fresh fruit, ¾ cup juice,*
½ cup canned or cooked fruit

FOOD GROUP: DAIRY PRODUCTS
Recommended servings: (optional) up to 3
Serving Sizes: *1 cup low-fat or nonfat milk or yogurt,*
1½ oz low-fat cheese

FOOD GROUP: EGGS
Recommended servings: (optional) limit to 3–4 yolks per week
Serving Sizes: *1 egg or 2 egg whites*

FOOD GROUP: FATS, SWEETS, AND ALCOHOL
Recommended servings: Go easy on all of these foods and beverages

---

Athletes may also be told that amino acids do not need to be digested before absorption and so replenish the body's proteins faster than the amino acids from high-protein foods. There is no evidence that more rapid absorption is beneficial—it takes hours, not minutes, to rebuild muscle proteins damaged during intense exercise.

A further claim for amino acid supplements is that they provide all the amino acids provided by food but are less taxing to the body's digestive system. Actually, the body quite readily produces an array of digestive enzymes that systematically break down the protein in food to amino acids before absorption.

Amino acid supplements usually contain only 200–500 milligrams of amino acids per capsule. On the other hand, 1 oz of beef, chicken, or fish supplies 7 gm of protein, which corresponds to 7,000 mg of amino acids! Thus, dietary sources of protein such as chicken or beans are in fact a "time release" source of amino acids.

The branched-chain amino acids—leucine, isoleucine, and valine—are the primary amino acids broken down for energy during prolonged endurance exercise. These amino acids are important nitrogen sources for the amino acid alanine, which is converted to glucose to help fuel endurance exercise. Because it is easy to obtain adequate quantities of branched-chain amino acids from food, endurance athletes don't require supplements.

PROBLEMS WITH HIGH-PROTEIN DIETS AND SUPPLEMENTS

Athletes who eat sufficient calories and obtain 12–15% of their calories from protein don't need protein supplements. The average diet already provides ample protein for muscle growth and repair. There is no evidence that protein supplements enhance muscle development, strength, or endurance. Extra protein doesn't help and may hurt health and performance.

The body can't tell the difference between protein obtained from food and protein obtained from expensive protein supplements. When athletes eat more protein than they require, the excess protein is either burned for energy or converted to fat, which many athletes don't realize. Burning protein for energy is expensive and wasteful. Carbohydrates are a more effective and less costly source of energy.

Consuming too much protein, whether from food or supplements, increases the body's water requirement and may contribute to dehydration. This is because the kidneys need more water to eliminate the excessive nitrogen load imposed by a high-protein intake. Athletes on high-protein diets should be sure to drink additional fluids to avoid becoming dehydrated.

High-protein diets are also usually high in fat. Consuming a high-protein, high-fat diet after heavy training will cause incomplete replacement of muscle glycogen and so impair performance. This type of diet also takes a long time to digest and can contribute to feeling sluggish. By comparison, a high-carbohydrate diet is easily digested and quickly restores muscle glycogen.

Keep in mind that high-fat diets can also increase the risk of health problems (more on this in the next chapter). Athletes on a high-protein diet should emphasize protein sources that are low in fat (nonfat dry milk powder, tuna in water, and beans). Chapter 12 provides guidelines on how to gain weight effectively.

Athletes who are determined to take protein supplements can use nonfat dry milk powder. It is a high-quality, inexpensive protein supplement (¼ cup provides 11 gm of protein) without the unproven additives such as chromium and amino acids that many protein or "weight gainer" supplements contain. Chapter 17 discusses the effectiveness of popular nutrition supplements.

There may be unidentified long-term risks associated with amino acid supplementation. Large intakes of some amino acids may interfere with the absorption of certain essential amino acids. When the body's proportion of amino acids is unbalanced, or if an essential amino acid is missing, the body can actually lose protein.

Taking ornithine supplements can cause mild to severe stomach cramping and diarrhea. Other amino acids alter nerve transmission in the brain. Some, such as methionine, are very toxic. Last, substituting amino acid supplements for food may cause deficiencies of other nutrients found in protein-rich foods, such as iron, niacin, and thiamin.

There is no evidence that supplementation with specific amino acids will increase muscle mass, decrease body fat, or improve endurance. It makes no sense for athletes to consume a product that has not been proved safe or effective, particularly when that product is promoted by people who stand to gain financially.

7

FAT:
FRIEND OR
ENEMY?

MANY PEOPLE ARE REDUCING their overall fat intake and watching the types of fat they eat to improve their health. Athletes need to be concerned about this as well, since exercise doesn't completely eliminate the health dangers of a high-fat diet.

Limiting fat in the diet is also beneficial for weight control. Fat is the most concentrated source of calories in the diet, supplying twice as many calories by weight as carbohydrate or protein. Dietary fat is also more readily converted to body fat than dietary carbohydrate.

This chapter discusses the importance of fat as a fuel, the health concerns of fat, ways to cut down on fat intake, and how high-fat diets affect performance. Misconceptions regarding exercise and body fat loss are also addressed.

IMPORTANCE OF FAT AS AN EXERCISE FUEL

Whereas the total glycogen stores in the muscle and liver amount to only 2,000 calories, every pound of fat supplies 3,500 calories. Fat is a major fuel for light- to moderate-intensity exercise.

Even though fat makes significant energy contributions during prolonged endurance exercise, athletes shouldn't attempt to increase their body fat stores. Even the leanest athletes have more body fat stored than they'll ever need. Excess body fat also impairs athletic performance.

Remember that endurance training increases the utilization of fat as fuel. The ability to use fat will spare muscle glycogen. This is advantageous during prolonged exercise since muscle glycogen depletion limits performance. Because muscle glycogen is limited and fat stores are abundant, slowing the rate of glycogen usage improves performance in endurance events such as marathons, bicycle road races, and triathlons.

Caffeine

Consuming 5–9 mg of caffeine per kg prior to endurance exercise may enhance performance by sparing muscle glycogen. Caffeine raises epinephrine (adrenaline) levels, which stimulate the release of free fatty acids from the adipose tissue. This increases fat utilization and reduces muscle glycogen usage.

However, the use of caffeine is considered a form of doping by the International Olympic Committee (IOC). The IOC has set an upper limit of 12 micrograms per milliliter of caffeine in the urine, which can be reached by consuming 800 milligrams of caffeine. Table 7-1 lists some common sources of caffeine. The pros and cons of this practice are discussed in Chapter 17.

FAT AND HEALTH

Americans typically eat an average of 37% of their total calories as fat. This high-fat diet increases the risk of developing heart disease (our nation's number one killer), stroke, and certain cancers. A high-fat diet also contributes to obesity, which is associated with a wide range of health problems.

TABLE 7-1
Sources of Caffeine

COFFEE (5-OZ CUP)		DRUGS (PER TABLET)	
Espresso	*150 mg*	**Pain Relievers**	
Drip	*110–150 mg*	*Excedrin*	*64–130 mg*
Percolator	*64–124 mg*	*Anacin, Emprin,*	
Instant	*40–108 mg*	*or Vanquish*	*32 mg*
Decaffeinated (instant)	*2 mg*	*Aspirin (plain)*	*0 mg*
Decaffeinated (brewed)	*2–5 mg*		
		Feminine Needs	
SOFT DRINKS (12 OUNCES)		*Pre Mens Forte*	*100 mg*
Diet Mr. Pibb	*59 mg*	*Pre Mens*	*66 mg*
Mountain Dew	*54 mg*	*Midol*	*32–65 mg*
Tab	*47 mg*		
Coca-Cola, Diet Coke	*46 mg*	**Diuretic**	
Shasta Cola, Diet Cola	*44 mg*	*Aqua-Ban*	*200 mg*
Shasta Cherry Cola	*44 mg*	*Permathene*	*200 mg*
Shasta Diet Cherry Cola	*44 mg*		
Sunkist Orange	*42 mg*	**Diet / Weight Control**	
Dr. Pepper	*40 mg*	*Dexatrim*	*200 mg*
Sugar-free Dr. Pepper	*40 mg*	*Dietac*	*200 mg*
Pepsi	*38 mg*	*Prolamine*	*140 mg*
Diet Pepsi, Pepsi Light	*36 mg*		
Royal Crown Cola	*36 mg*	**Alertness/Stimulants**	
Diet Rite	*36 mg*	*Vivarin*	*200 mg*
		NoDoz	*100–200mg*
TEA (5-OZ CUP)			
Black tea brewed 5 min	*20–50 mg*		
Black tea brewed 3 min	*20–46 mg*		
Black tea brewed 1 min	*9–33 mg*		
Green tea	*30 mg*		
Instant tea	*12–28 mg*		
Ice tea (12-oz can)	*22–36 mg*		

✔ **Note:** Products change from time to time, and caffeine content may also change.
■ **Source:** *Maximize Your Body Potential*, by Joyce D. Nash, Ph.D., Bull Publishing Company, Palo Alto, CA. Used with permission.

Athletes, as all Americans, should consume less than 30% of their total calories from fat and limit cholesterol to 300 mg/day. Because saturated fat increases the cholesterol level in the blood, it should provide less than 10% of total calories. An elevated blood cholesterol level is a major risk factor for heart disease, as are smoking, high blood pressure, and inactivity.

The National Cholesterol Education Program defines a desirable blood cholesterol level as below 200 mg/dL. A blood cholesterol level of 240 mg/dL or more is considered high, and 200–239 mg/dL is considered borderline high. These levels are significant, as a cholesterol level of 240 mg/dL doubles the risk of heart disease compared to a cholesterol level of 200 mg/dL.

How cholesterol is transported in the blood also affects the risk of developing heart disease. Cholesterol is transported in the blood attached to protein as a substance called a lipoprotein. Low-density lipoprotein (LDL) is the main component of the total cholesterol level. LDL deposits cholesterol in the artery wall and increases the risk of heart disease. High-density lipoprotein (HDL), on the other hand, removes cholesterol from the artery wall and actually decreases the risk of heart disease.

An LDL cholesterol level below 130 mg/dL is considered desirable, as shown in Table 7-2. A level of 130–159 mg/dL is considered borderline high, and a level of 160 mg/dL is considered high. A high level of HDL cholesterol is protective against heart disease, and levels of 60 mg/dL or above significantly decrease heart disease risk. On the other hand, a low level of HDL cholesterol (less than 35 mg/dL) significantly increases the risk of developing heart disease.

In general, decreasing the intake of saturated fat and cholesterol lowers LDL cholesterol levels and regular exercise raises HDL cholesterol levels.

CUTTING DOWN ON FAT INTAKE

You can obtain a high-carbohydrate, low-fat diet by following the training diet guidelines outlined in Chapter 2. Here are further recommendations to cut down on fat intake:

Athletes can lower their fat intake by cutting down on both "hidden" and "visible" sources of fat, as shown in Table 7-3 (page 70). Fat is hidden in dairy products, meat, eggs, nuts, and fried foods. Be aware of the hidden fat in favorite foods such as ice cream, cheese, french fries, chips, granola, cold cuts, bacon,

---

TABLE 7-2
It Pays to Know Your Blood Cholesterol Level

BLOOD CHOLESTEROL LEVEL (MG/DL)

< (less than) 200 ....*Desirable level*
200–239 ....*Borderline-high level*
> (more than) 239 ....*High level*

RECOMMENDED FOLLOW-UP

Total cholesterol < 200 mg/dL	*Repeat within 5 years*
Total cholesterol 200–239 mg/dL *Without existent heart disease* *or 2 heart-disease risk factors*	*Blood cholesterol rechecked annually*
With 2 other heart-disease risk factors	*Lipoprotein analysis:* *further action based on LDL cholesterol level*
Total cholesterol > 239mg/dL, *regardless of other factors*	*Same as for previous group*

LDL CHOLESTEROL LEVELS (MG/DL)

< 130 ....*Desirable level*
130–159 ....*Borderline-high level*
> 159 ....*High-risk level*

RISK FACTORS FOR HEART DISEASE
Positive Risk Factors
Age
- *Male ≥ 45 years*
- *Female ≥ 55 years or early menopause without estrogen-replacement therapy*
- *Family history of premature heart disease (definite myocardial infarction or sudden death before 55 years of age in father or before 65 years of age in mother)*
- *Current cigarette smoking*
- *Hypertension (≥ 140/90 mm Hg or on blood pressure medication)*
- *Low HDL cholesterol (< 35 mg/dL)*
- *Diabetes*

Negative Risk Factor
High HDL cholesterol (≥ 60 mg/dL)

---

nuts, hamburger, and baked goods (cookies, pies, cakes, and pastries). Visible dietary sources of fat include margarine, butter, cream, mayonnaise, oil, salad dressing, gravies, sauces, sour cream, and cream cheese.

TABLE 7-3
Recommended Diet Modifications to Lower Blood Cholesterol

	CHOOSE	DECREASE
Fish, Chicken, Turkey, and Lean Meats	*Fish, poultry without skin, lean cuts of beef, lamb, pork or veal, shellfish*	*Fatty cuts of beef, lamb, pork; spare ribs, organ meats, regular cold cuts, sausage, hot dogs, bacon, sardines, roe*
Skim and Low-fat Milk, Cheese Yogurt, and Dairy Substitutes	*Skim or 1% fat milk (liquid, powdered, evaporated), buttermilk*	*Whole milk (4% fat): regular, evaporated, condensed; cream, half and half, 2% milk, imitation milk products, most nondairy creamers, whipped toppings*
	Nonfat (0% fat) or low-fat yogurt	*Whole-milk yogurt*
	Low-fat cottage cheese (1% or 2% fat)	*Whole-milk cottage cheese (4% fat)*
	Low-fat cheeses, farmer, or pot cheeses (all of these should be labeled no more than 2–6 gm fat/ounce)	*All natural cheeses (e.g., blue, roquefort, camembert, cheddar, swiss)*
		Low-fat or "Light" cream cheese, low-fat or "Light" sour cream Cream cheeses, sour cream
	Sherbet Sorbet	*Ice cream*
Eggs	*Egg whites (2 whites equals 1 whole egg in recipes), cholesterol-free egg substitutes*	*Egg yolks*
Fruits and Vegetables	*Fresh, frozen, canned, or dried fruits and vegetables*	*Vegetables prepared in butter, cream, or other sauces*
Breads and Cereals	*Homemade baked goods using unsaturated oils sparingly, angel food cake, low-fat crackers, low-fat cookies*	*Commercial baked goods: pies, cakes, donuts, croissants, pastries, muffins, biscuits, high-fat crackers, high-fat cookies*
	Rice, pasta	*Egg noodles*

TABLE 7-3 (continued)
Recommended Diet Modifications to Lower Blood Cholesterol

	CHOOSE	DECREASE
Breads and Cereals (continued)	*Whole-grain breads and cereals (oatmeal, whole wheat, rye, bran, multigrain, etc.)*	*Breads in which eggs are major ingredient*
Fats and Oils	*Baking cocoa*	*Chocolate*
	Unsaturated vegetable oils: corn, olive, rapeseed (canola oil), safflower, sesame, soybean, sunflower	*Butter, coconut oil, palm oil, palm kernel oil, lard, bacon fat*
	Tub margarine or shortening made from one of the unsaturated oils listed above	*Stick margarine*
	Diet margarine	
	Mayonnaise, salad dressings made with unsaturated oils listed above	*Dressings made with egg yolk*
	Low-fat dressings	*Regular dressings*
	Seeds and nuts	*Coconut*

The intake of total fat, saturated fat, and cholesterol can be reduced by choosing lean meat, poultry, and fish. High-fat processed meat such as bologna, bacon, salami, and hot dogs should be eaten sparingly. Removing the skin from poultry and trimming visible fat from meat also cuts down on fat. The Dietary Guidelines for Americans recommend limiting the consumption of meat, poultry, and fish to about 6 ounces per day.

The butterfat found in butter, cheese, chocolate, ice cream, and whole milk should also be limited to reduce the intake of total fat, saturated fat, and cholesterol. Nonfat and low-fat dairy products such as 1% fat milk and yogurt, ice milk, and low-fat cheese can be substituted for high-fat dairy products. The Dietary Guidelines recommend consuming two to three servings of dairy products each day.

Oils with high percentages of unsaturated fat (canola, corn, olive and soy oil, and their derivative margarines) should be substituted for saturated fats such as butter, lard, shortening, and bacon grease. When oil and margarine are substituted for butter, keep in mind that they are still high in fat and calories and should be used sparingly. Nonfat substitutes for salad dressing and sour cream can replace the regular higher-fat versions. Although nonfat and low-fat products contain little or no fat, they do contain calories. Remember to check the food label—fat free does not mean calorie free. These products can be loaded with extra sodium and sugar to improve taste, as shown in Table 7-4.

Choose cooking methods that require little or no fat. These include steaming, baking, broiling, grilling, poaching, or stir-frying in small amounts of unsaturated vegetable oil. Foods can be microwaved or cooked using sprays to coat pans to reduce added fat. Limit fried foods, especially when saturated fat is used.

FAT AND PERFORMANCE

High-fat diets are sometimes promoted to improve performance in endurance events. The claim is that "fat loading" enables the athlete to burn fat, rather than glycogen, as the major fuel source. Because fat stores are plentiful and glycogen stores are limited, fat loading supposedly enhances endurance.

There is no convincing evidence that high-fat diets increase endurance. In fact, just the opposite is likely to occur. Eating too much fat will decrease the intake of carbohydrate. Muscle glycogen stores cannot be adequately maintained on a high-fat diet. Muscle glycogen is the preferred fuel for high-intensity exercise because fat breakdown can't supply energy fast enough. Most endurance athletes train and compete at an intensity that requires carbohydrate for fuel. The bottom line: Performance will be impaired on a high-fat diet.

TABLE 7-4
A Matter of Fat

FOOD	AMOUNT	CALORIES	FAT (gm)	CARBOHYDRATE (gm)
Strawberry danish	*1 slice*	220	12	27
Fat-free strawberry danish	*1 slice*	140	0	33
Creme cookie	*3 cookies*	173	8.25	24
Low-fat creme cookie	*3 cookies*	165	3.75	32

The other drawbacks of high-fat diets outweigh any potential benefits. Such diets need medical supervision—they have been associated with sudden death and heart rhythm disturbances due to protein and potassium losses.

The blood cholesterol level can rise on a high-fat diet despite heavy training. Because exercise by itself doesn't prevent heart disease, eating a high-fat diet for a long time may increase the athlete's risk of acquiring heart disease.

A high-fat diet takes longer to digest, which is one of the reasons fat should be limited in the pre-exercise meal. Examples of "fat loading" meals include cheese, marbled or ground beef, eggs, butter, and tuna mixed with mayonnaise. A diet of such foods lacks the variety of nutrients needed for optimal performance.

Adapting to a high-fat diet takes at least two weeks. During this time, exercising will be difficult and unpleasant due to low muscle glycogen stores. Even after adaptation is complete, the athlete won't be able to sustain the intensity required for most endurance competitions.

It makes no sense for endurance athletes to try to adjust to a high-fat diet when they can get the immediate performance benefits of a high-carbohydrate diet. The ability to burn fat is increased more effectively by endurance training than by eating a high-fat diet. In any case, the harmful health effects of high-fat diets make them too risky for endurance athletes.

EXERCISE AND BODY FAT LOSS

It is well known that fat makes its greatest energy contribution during low- to moderate-intensity exercise. This has led to recommendations that individuals who want to lose weight should exercise at a lower intensity.

The concept of "fat burning" versus "carbohydrate burning" exercises is a common misconception. Some believe that individuals who want to lose body fat should exercise at a lower intensity since fat contributes more to the metabolic mixture. Unfortunately, this assumption misses the whole point: Regular exercise is beneficial for weight loss because it creates a prolonged caloric deficit.

The fuel being burned to create this caloric deficit (fat or carbohydrate) is not important. There is no scientific evidence that using fat as fuel will produce greater body fat loss than using carbohydrate as fuel. It is the caloric deficit produced that is important.

For example, it is doubtful that a runner would lose more body fat by jogging five miles slowly than by running five miles at race pace. Although fat contributes more calories during jogging than racing, both activities burn the same amount of calories and so have the same effect on body fat.

Although a greater percentage of fat may be burned with low-intensity exercise, the total amount of fat burned is actually greater with high-intensity exercise because the total energy expenditure is higher during intense activity. The fuel burned during exercise (carbohydrate or fat) doesn't matter when the goal is to lose weight.

In other words, low-intensity exercise uses a greater percentage of fat than high-intensity exercise, but the fat calories (and carbohydrate calories) are being burned at a relatively slow rate —4 to 5 calories per minute.

By comparison, high-intensity exercise uses a smaller percentage of fat, but this smaller percentage (along with carbohydrate) is burned at a much higher rate—10 to 15 calories per minute. So, the total amount of fat burned is greater at the higher-intensity levels.

Many individuals have confused the proportion of fat used as fuel with the more important rate of fuel utilization, which is a key concept in exercise-induced body fat loss. When the goal of an exercise program is to lose weight, the exercise should create a caloric deficit. To lose 1 pound of body fat, an individual must expend 3,500 calories, whether those calories come from fat or from carbohydrate.

The person's fitness level must be considered when exercise is recommended as part of a weight-loss program. Low- to moderate-intensity exercise is recommended for overweight people who are just starting to exercise. High-intensity exercise is associated with an increased risk of orthopedic injuries. Also, unfit people who engage in high-intensity exercise usually find it unpleasant and may stop exercising altogether.

Individuals who are just starting to exercise for weight loss should exercise at a lower intensity. The only drawback of low-intensity exercise is that the person must exercise longer to achieve a significant caloric deficit. Other than that, a low-intensity workout that expends 300 calories in 1 hour is just as beneficial for body fat loss as a high-intensity workout that expends 300 calories in 30 minutes.

Keep in mind that the decreased number of calories burned during low-intensity exercise may be detrimental for fit people trying to lose body fat. If the fit person's food intake stays the same and the exercise time isn't increased to compensate for the reduced caloric expenditure of low-intensity exercise, the result may be a slow but steady weight gain!

8

VITAMINS AND MINERALS: HELP OR HYPE?

NUMEROUS ADVERTISEMENTS CLAIM that athletes and active people require large doses or special mixtures of vitamins and minerals to support their active lifestyles. The Food and Drug Administration estimates that about 40% of all Americans rely on self-prescribed vitamin and mineral supplements. Athletes, coaches, and athletic trainers are favorite targets of the supplement salespeople.

Many athletes assume that if a small amount of a nutrient is good, more will be better. In addition to seeking a competitive edge, athletes may feel that their diets are inadequate and so take supplements for "nutritional insurance."

In small amounts, vitamins function as catalysts—substances that increase the speed of a reaction without being used up by the reaction. The fact that vitamins aren't used up explains why they are needed only in small amounts.

Contrary to popular belief, vitamins do not provide energy, although some vitamins *are* important for the release of energy

FIGURE 8-1
The B Vitamins
The B vitamins are important for the release of energy from carbohydrate in the muscle cell.

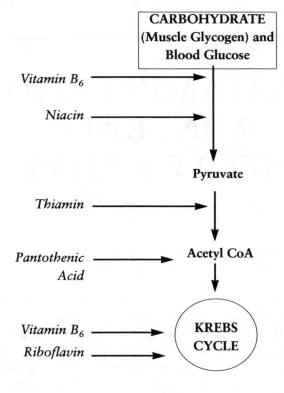

from carbohydrate (see Figure 8-1). Only protein, carbohydrate, and fat provide energy (calories). This means that in general the vitamin requirements of an active person are not greater than those of a sedentary person. Thiamin, riboflavin, and niacin are an exception, because they are required in proportion to calories consumed and active people need more calories. However, a balanced diet provides ample amounts of these vitamins. It is supplied by those carbohydrate-rich foods recommended for athletes—bread and whole-grain or enriched-grain products.

This chapter discusses the importance of the recommended dietary allowances for vitamins and minerals, supplementation concerns, and supplement recommendations. Iron and calcium are minerals of specific concern for women and are addressed in Chapter 13. The antioxidant vitamins—vitamins C, E, and beta-carotene—have received a lot of attention recently and are also discussed here.

RECOMMENDED DIETARY ALLOWANCES

The National Academy of Sciences has established and regularly updates recommended dietary allowances (RDAs) as a guide for determining nutritional needs. The RDA is an amount of an essential nutrient that is scientifically judged to be adequate to meet the known nutrient needs of practically all healthy people.

The RDA is not the smallest amount required to prevent disease symptoms, since a large margin of safety is included. For example, the body requires about 10 milligrams of vitamin C daily to prevent the deficiency disease scurvy, but the RDA for vitamin C is set at 60 milligrams.

Many athletes feel that taking vitamin/mineral supplements is justified because the RDAs don't account for the varying nutritional needs of different people. In general, the nutrient needs for the average person are only about two-thirds of the RDA. This means that as long as athletes consume at least 67% of the RDA for a given nutrient, they are probably protected from a nutritional deficiency.

As a further example, the RDA for vitamins varies only slightly among different ages, sizes, and sexes. Generally, a large active man doesn't require significantly more vitamins than a small sedentary woman. Even during the most demanding nutritional situations such as pregnancy and breast-feeding, the increased need for vitamins is modest.

SUPPLEMENTATION CONCERNS

High doses of vitamins (amounts 10 times the RDA for water-soluble vitamins, 5 times the RDA for fat-soluble vitamins) can be dangerous. When vitamins are taken in such huge amounts, they no longer function as vitamins—they become drugs and may produce serious side effects.

As mentioned in Chapter 1, fat-soluble vitamins (A and D in particular) can build up in the body to toxic levels. Large doses of water-soluble vitamins can also cause side effects. Some body builders take large doses of niacin (a B vitamin) to make their blood vessels dilate and stand out. However, large amounts of niacin can cause severe flushing, skin disorders, liver damage, ulcers, and blood sugar disorders. High doses of niacin also interfere with fat metabolism and speed up glycogen depletion.

Niacin may be useful in the treatment of elevated blood cholesterol and triglycerides, but it should *never* be used for this purpose without medical supervision. Large doses of vitamin C have been associated with diarrhea, kidney stone formation, and impaired copper absorption.

Vitamin B_6 (pyridoxine) toxicity has been documented in women who have taken supplements to alleviate premenstrual symptoms. Excess vitamin B_6 can cause neurological symptoms similiar to multiple sclerosis, including numbness and tingling of the hands, difficulty in walking, and electric shocks shooting down the spine. Toxicity has been reported in people taking as little as 200 milligrams a day—the RDA for vitamin B_6 is about 2 milligrams.

Like excess amounts of fat-soluble vitamins, excess amounts of minerals are stored in the body and can gradually build up to toxic levels. An excess of one mineral can interfere with the functioning of others. Since iron overload can damage the liver, pancreas, and heart, it should be used only for proven iron deficiency. While about 6% of Americans are iron deficient and will benefit from iron supplementation, more than 10% of Americans have excess iron in their bodies and can be harmed by iron supplementation.

Athletes often feel that their "run-down feeling" is due to a vitamin or mineral deficiency. When there is a nutritional reason for fatigue, it is usually an inadequate intake of calories, carbohydrate, or dehydration. Athletes who are always tired may be eating too little carbohydrate or calories for glycogen synthesis, or they may be overtraining. When people feel better after taking vitamin/mineral supplements, it's probably due to the strength of their belief that the supplements help—the placebo effect.

Supplementation at levels exceeding the RDA does not improve the performance of well-nourished athletes. Although vitamin and mineral deficiencies can impair athletic performance, it's very unusual for active people to have such deficiencies. There is a close relationship between caloric intake and vitamin intake: The more food eaten, the greater the vitamin and mineral intake. Athletes generally eat more than sedentary people and so tend to get more vitamins and minerals in relation to their needs. Also, a diet high in complex carbohydrates—the recommended diet for athletes—contains foods with a variety of nutrients.

SUPPLEMENT RECOMMENDATIONS

Does anyone need vitamin/mineral supplements? The Council on Scientific Affairs of the American Medical Association (AMA) has published a report on the appropriate use of supplements. This report states that healthy adult men and women who aren't pregnant or breast-feeding do not require supplements—provided that they're eating a balanced and varied diet.

The Council concedes that, due to changing dietary habits (increased consumption of processed and fast foods), there may be instances where vitamin intake is inadequate. Before opting for supplementation, however, you should attempt to improve your food selection and eating habits.

Supplements containing 2 to 10 times the RDA should be considered therapeutic and used only under medical supervision. In such cases, the supplement is used to treat specific disease states or conditions that limit the absorption of a specific vitamin or which increase the requirement for it.

The Committee on Diet and Health (Food and Nutrition Board, National Research Council) recommends that people avoid taking dietary supplements that exceed 100% of the RDA in any one day. Most people can, and should, obtain essential nutrients from a variety of foods.

The Committee noted possible exceptions in the cases of women who are pregnant or breast-feeding, women with excess monthly bleeding, people on very-low-calorie diets, some vegetarians, and people with malabsorption problems. However, rather than automatically taking vitamin/mineral supplements, these individuals should be evaluated on a case-by-case basis.

Athletes who limit their caloric intake are also at risk for nutritional deficiencies. These include athletes who are concerned about how extra weight affects performance or cosmetics. Often these are athletes competing in long-distance running, gymnastics, dancing, figure skating, and diving and those who are required to "make weight"—wrestlers, boxers, and weight-classified football or crew participants. Weight-conscious casual athletes may also be at risk. A vitamin/mineral supplement supplying no more than 100% of the RDA might be appropriate for some of these individuals.

For active people and athletes who do not fall into any of these categories, most health authorities agree that there is no harm in a simple vitamin/mineral supplement, provided that it does not exceed 100% of the RDA for nutrients. Keep in mind there is also no evidence that this supplementation is beneficial.

The AMA Council condemns the increasing use of megadose vitamin/mineral therapy because it is based on anecdotal, nonscientific evidence. Megadose therapy only thins wallets and builds false hopes, without providing any beneficial results. More important, the consumption of large amounts of vitamins and minerals can produce toxic effects and/or upset the delicate balance of these nutrients.

It's much easier to take vitamin/mineral supplements than to change eating habits. Supplements provide the illusion of caring for health but remove the responsibility of dietary change. Performance can't be improved simply by taking a pill. Just as a balanced diet isn't improved by supplements, an inadequate diet isn't "fixed" by supplements.

By eating a variety of high-quality foods from the Food Guide Pyramid each day, you eliminate the need for vitamin/mineral supplements. Athletes who desire nutritional insurance can eat more complex carbohydrates and fewer empty calories (sugar, fat, and alcohol).

ANTIOXIDANTS

Some athletes take antioxidant supplements—vitamins C, E, and beta-carotene—believing that this will reduce the amount of muscle damage caused by heavy exercise. Antioxidant supplements are promoted as protection against serious conditions such as heart disease, cancer, and even the aging process.

Free radicals, substances that can damage muscle cells and cell membranes, are released by the body's own normal process of producing energy. The production of free radicals can also be increased by exposure to various environmental pollutants such as smog, cigarette smoke, radiation, and certain pesticides.

Fortunately, the body possesses its own antioxidant defense of enzymes and nutrients such as vitamins E, C, and beta-carotene. Each of these antioxidants works at different sites within the body and in a unique way. Their overall goal, however, is to stop the production and spread of harmful free-radical chain reactions.

Exercise causes a number of physiological changes that increase the production of free radicals. These include an elevated metabolic rate, increased body temperature, and higher epinephrine levels. Considering this, it's not surprising that some athletes believe that antioxidant supplements might protect against exercise-induced muscle damage.

Regular physical training itself provides a partially protective effect for athletes. Consistent workouts increase the activity of the enzymes that clean up the free radicals, thereby helping to minimize muscle damage.

Though antioxidant supplements may protect against muscle damage, they won't help the performance of adequately nourished athletes. For example, vitamin E deficiency does impair endurance capacity and this is associated with greater free-radical damage. However, vitamin E supplementation doesn't improve aerobic capacity or endurance in well-nourished athletes.

The decision about whether or not to take antioxidant supplements is difficult, based on the current state of research. The RDAs of 60 mg of vitamin C, 30 IU (international units) of vitamin E, and 6 mg of beta-carotene can be readily obtained through diet. In the small quantities found in food, these nutrients help to stop the production and spread of harmful free-radical chain reactions.

There is a risk that in the high amounts found in supplements, vitamins C, E, and beta-carotene may actually *increase* the production of free radicals. Antioxidant supplements have *not* been proved to do more good than harm, which is why the Food and Drug Administration won't permit them to be marketed with claims that they can prevent disease.

Regardless of supplements, all athletes will benefit from consuming the recommended amount of vegetables (three to four servings) and fruit (two to four servings) a day, as these foods contain antioxidant vitamins in addition to other important nutrients.

Athletes should avoid taking large doses of the minerals that work with the free-radical suppressing enzymes—zinc, copper, and selenium. Excess zinc consumption may reduce HDL cholesterol levels, impair immune function, and inhibit copper absorption from foods, possibly leading to anemia. Copper supplements aren't recommended since athletes don't appear to be deficient and there's no evidence to suggest that copper will enhance performance.

Selenium is a particular supplement favorite, because it works with vitamin E to protect cell membranes against free-radical damage. However, research suggests that vitamin E, rather than selenium, is crucial for protection against free-radical damage. There is no reason to take selenium supplements as most people get enough selenium from their diet and an excess intake may be harmful.

9

FLUID
REQUIREMENTS
AND HYDRATION

WATER IS THE MOST ESSENTIAL of all nutrients since the body requires it constantly. All of the body's important chemical reactions, such as energy production, are carried out in water. Without water, most people could not survive for more than a few days. Although water has a number of important functions, the most critical function for athletes is the regulation of body temperature.

This chapter discusses the distribution of water in the body, the importance of water for temperature regulation during exercise, heat illnesses, and fluid needs of athletes. Then fluid-replacement beverages and the role of electrolytes (sodium and potassium) are examined. Last, the effects of alcoholic and caffeinated beverages on performance are addressed.

DISTRIBUTION OF BODY WATER

Water is stored in several areas of the body but moves continually between these areas. About 65% of the body's water is stored inside the cells as intracellular water. The remaining 35% is stored outside the cells as extracellular water. The extracellular water is divided into the interstitial water between or surrounding the cells and the vascular water within the circulating blood.

Proper water and electrolyte balance within these areas is extremely important for athletes. Fluid shifts such as decreases in the blood volume and cellular dehydration can occur from sweat losses during exercise in the heat. Dehydration contributes to fatigue and increases the risk of developing heat illnesses.

Water makes up about 60% of the body weight in the average adult male and about 50% in the adult female. This percentage may be as low as 40% in obese individuals and as high as 70% in muscular ones. This difference in water content is due to the fact that fat tissue is low in water (about 10–15%) and muscle tissue is high in water (about 70–75%). Thus, athletes who have a high muscle mass and low fat content have a relatively high body water content.

WATER AND TEMPERATURE REGULATION DURING EXERCISE

Water acts as a coolant to keep the body from overheating during physical activity. During exercise, heat is generated as a by-product of the working muscles. When heat builds up, the body temperature rises. This heat must be removed to maintain a normal body temperature.

During exercise in warm weather, sweat is the body's main mechanism for getting rid of excess heat. When sweat evaporates from the skin, the body cools down. Large sweat losses, however, reduce the body's water content. The loss of water in sweat harms athletic performance and hinders the body's ability to control body temperature. Here's why:

During exercise in the heat, blood that was transferring oxygen to the muscles is diverted to skin to help eliminate heat. The competition for blood between the muscles and skin places a greater demand on the cardiovascular system. This is happening at a time when the blood volume is decreasing due to sweat losses.

The fluid in sweat initially comes from the extracellular fluid compartments: the blood plasma and the interstitial fluid. Eventually, intracellular fluid will also be reduced as the increase in extracellular sodium levels draws water from the intracellular space. It is interesting that the muscle and skin contribute about 70% of the total water lost in sweat, which may protect the brain and other vital organs.

The body is programmed to protect cardiovascular function at the expense of body temperature regulation. Consequently, skin blood flow and sweat rate are decreased in an effort to conserve body fluid. As a result, the body temperature rises, leading to fatigue and increased risk of heat injury.

In practical terms, when you're dehydrated you can't exercise as hard or as long. During prolonged exercise in the heat, sweat losses constituting as little as 2% of your body weight impair athletic performance and temperature regulation. Inadequate fluid replacement speeds up dehydration and can ultimately cause a life-threatening heat illness.

WEATHER CONCERNS

Athletes may be unaware of the enormous sweat losses that can occur during hot, dry weather. Large amounts of fluid evaporate very quickly in these conditions. Because athletes don't feel sweaty, they may not recognize how much water they've lost.

Besides heat, relative humidity is important. As the moisture in the air increases, the effectiveness of heat loss through sweating decreases. If the air is saturated with water, little evaporation will occur even at cooler temperatures and body heat can build up. Conversely, when the sweat "drips" off the skin, the person is not getting the cooling benefit of sweat. Athletes should be aware of intense physical exertion on warm, humid days, as well as on hot, dry days (see Table 9-1).

TABLE 9-1
Heat Index

TEMPERATURE

Relative Humidity	70°	75°	80°	85°	90°	95°	100°	105°	110°	115°	120°
						Apparent Temperature*					
0%	64°	69°	73°	78°	83°	87°	91°	95°	99°	103°	107°
10%	65°	70°	75°	80°	85°	90°	95°	100°	105°	111°	116°
20%	66°	72°	77°	82°	87°	93°	99°	105°	112°	120°	130°
30%	67°	73°	78°	84°	90°	96°	104°	113°	123°	135°	148°
40%	68°	74°	79°	86°	93°	101°	110°	123°	137°	151°	
50%	69°	75°	81°	88°	96°	107°	120°	135°	150°		
60%	70°	76°	82°	90°	100°	114°	132°	149°			
70%	70°	77°	85°	93°	106°	124°	144°				
80%	71°	78°	86°	97°	113°	136°					
90%	71°	79°	88°	102°	122°						
100%	72°	80°	91°	108°							

HOW TO USE HEAT INDEX:
1. Across top locate Temperature
2. Down left side locate Relative Humidity
3. Follow across and down to find Apparent Temperature
4. Determine Heat Stress Risk on chart below

Apparent Temperature	Heat Stress Risk with Physical Activity and/or Prolonged Exposure
90°–105°	*Heat cramps or heat exhaustion* possible
105°–130°	*Heat cramps or heat exhaustion* likely *Heatstroke* possible
130° and up	*Heatstroke* highly likely

✔ **Note:** *Combined index of heat and humidity. . . what it feels like to the body.
✔ **Note:** This heat index chart is designed to provide general guidelines for assessing the potential severity of heat stress. Individual reactions to heat will vary. In addition, studies indicate that susceptibility to heat disorders tends to increase with age. Exposure to full sunshine can increase Heat Index values by up to 15°F.
■ **Source:** National Oceanic and Atmospheric Administration.

To prevent problems caused by heat and humidity, exercise at the coolest time of the day. Avoid practice during the middle of the day when the temperature is usually the highest. If you must practice or compete then, gradually build up your tolerance to the heat. This can be accomplished by holding short workouts in the heat each day. Over time, the length of the workout can be slowly increased.

Clothing and sports gear also affect sweating and body temperature. Sweat suits and other heavy gear trap sweat and so prevent evaporation. This leads to a build-up of body heat. In hot or humid weather, wear the lightest clothing possible. Mesh jerseys, lightweight shorts, and low-cut socks allow more heat to evaporate than do sweat suits and heavy gear.

HEAT ILLNESSES

Athletes who don't exercise prudently in hot or humid weather can experience heat cramps, heat exhaustion, or heatstroke. Three factors contribute to the development of heat injuries: increased core temperature, loss of body fluids, and loss of electrolytes.

Heat Cramps

Heat cramps, or involuntary muscle spasms, occur during or after activity, usually in the specific muscles exercised. This form of heat illness is probably due to an imbalance of the body's fluid and electrolyte concentrations, as shown in Figure 9-1. Muscle spasms can occur if the electrolytes lost in sweat aren't replaced. Treatment: Rest, drink fluids with electrolytes such as sports drinks, and add salt to foods.

Heat Exhaustion

Heat exhaustion may be caused by a reduced blood volume due to excessive sweating. Blood then pools in the extremities and

FIGURE 9-1
Causes of Muscle Cramps

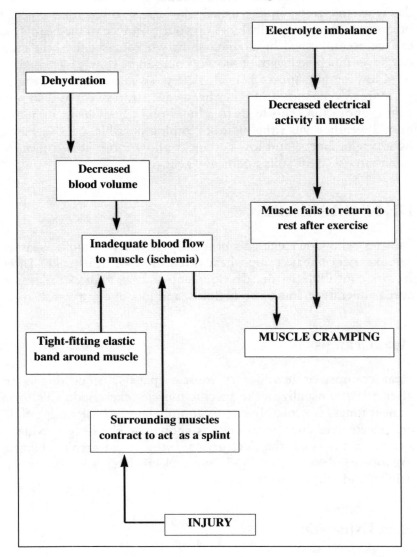

the athlete may faint or feel dizzy. The symptoms of heat exhaustion also include nausea and fatigue. Although sweating may be reduced, the athlete's rectal temperature is not elevated to dangerous levels (it remains lower than 104°F). Treatment: Rest in a cool place and drink fluids containing electrolytes. Medical attention may be required.

Heatstroke

Heatstroke is a medical emergency requiring immediate action. It occurs when the body's temperature-regulating processes simply stop functioning. Sweating usually stops and the skin becomes dry and hot. The athlete's rectal temperature is excessively high —over 105.8°F. Other symptoms include disorientation, vomiting, headache, and unconsciousness. If heatstroke is untreated, death occurs due to circulatory collapse and central nervous system damage. Treatment: Aggressive steps must be taken to immediately lower elevated body temperature. Until medical help arrives, the athlete can be covered with ice packs, immersed in cold water, or rubbed with alcohol.

Athletes must be aware of the symptoms of impending heat illness. These include weakness, feeling of chills, goose pimples on the chest and upper arms, nausea, headache, faintness, disorientation, muscle cramping, and cessation of sweating. Continuing to exercise when experiencing any of these symptoms can lead to a heat injury.

FLUID-REPLACEMENT GUIDELINES

At rest, athletes need between 2 and 3 quarts of fluid daily. Exercise greatly increases fluid requirements. Consuming cool fluids regularly during exercise protects your health and will optimize athletic performance. Proper hydration is the most frequently overlooked performance aid.

Athletes can prepare for exercise in the heat by drinking 8 to 16 ounces of rapidly absorbed fluid (water or sports drink) 15 minutes before exercise. This technique is called hyperhydration and helps to lower the body's core temperature and so reduce the added stress heat places on the cardiovascular system.

Drinking during exercise is essential to prevent the detrimental effects of dehydration on body temperature and exercise performance. As shown in Table 9-2, athletes should drink 4 to 8 ounces of rapidly absorbed fluid every 15 minutes during exercise. Obviously, the actual amount consumed during exercise will vary based on the rate of dehydration due to sweating.

There is no safe level of dehydration that can be tolerated before cardiovascular function and temperature regulation are impaired. Athletes will perform at their best when their fluid intake closely matches their fluid losses from sweating.

Thirst is not an adequate guide to fluid replacement, since athletes replace only 50% of their fluid losses during exercise. It's necessary to regulate fluid intake by drinking according to a time schedule rather than by perceived thirst.

Athletes need to get in the habit of regular drinking during training. Some athletes pay attention to their fluid intake only during competition and become dehydrated in practice sessions. Heat injury can occur just as easily during training. At the very least, dehydration impairs performance in practice. Adequate fluid consumption during training protects against heat illness and enables athletes to get the most out of their practice sessions. It also allows them to practice proper hydration techniques in preparation for competition.

Occasionally fluids are restricted during practice so that athletes won't "depend" on them during competition. Withholding fluids during practice won't make athletes better prepared for competition—it will increase their risk of heat injury. The body can't adapt to becoming dehydrated.

Athletes should weigh both before and after exercise (nude is best) to determine how much fluid they're losing. For every pound of body weight lost after exercise, the athlete should drink 16 ounces of fluid. If a gradual loss of weight is noticed during warm-

---

TABLE 9-2
Hydration Guidelines

- 8 to 16 ounces 15 minutes before exercise
- 4 to 8 ounces every 15 minutes during exercise
- 16 ounces for every pound of body weight lost after exercise

---

weather training, it may be due to chronic dehydration rather than body fat loss. Athletes can also check the color of their urine. Urine that is dark in color may indicate a dehydrated state.

FLUID-REPLACEMENT BEVERAGES

Athletes can consume water or a sports drink to replace fluid losses. Sports drinks containing carbohydrate and sodium such as Gatorade are absorbed as quickly as water. The presence of glucose and sodium in sports drinks increases fluid uptake in the small intestine. Table 9-3 lists some popular sports drinks.

Sports drinks promote optimal cardiovascular function and temperature regulation as well as plain water does. However, sports drinks improve performance during prolonged exercise by providing carbohydrate for the working muscles. For exercise lasting an hour or longer, sports drinks provide a performance edge that water can't. Sports drinks are also beneficial when you're exercising for an hour several times a day. However, water remains an effective and inexpensive fluid-replacement beverage for exercise lasting less than an hour.

For optimal absorption and performance, a sports drink should contain 6–8% carbohydrate—about 60 to 80 calories per 8 ounces. It is doubtful that drinks containing less than 5% carbohydrate, about 50 calories per 8 ounces, will help performance. Those that exceed 10% carbohydrate, about 100 calories per 8 ounces—fruit juices, sodas, and concentrated fructose drinks—take longer to be absorbed and can cause abdominal cramps, nausea, bloating, and diarrhea.

TABLE 9-3
Fluid Replacement Beverages

BEVERAGE	FLAVORS	CARBOHYDRATE INGREDIENT	CARBOHYDRATE %(CONCENTRATION) PER 8 OZ	SODIUM (MG) PER 8 OZ	POTASSIUM (MG)	OTHER MINERALS AND VITAMINS
Gatorade® Thirst Quencher The Gatorade Company	Lemon-lime, orange, fruit punch, lemonade, citrus cooler, tropical fruit, grape, iced tea cooler	Powder: sucrose and glucose; Liquid: Sucrose and glucose/syrup solids	6	110	30	Chloride, phosphorus
Powerade® Coca-Cola	Lemon-lime, fruit punch, orange, grape	High fructose corn syrup, maltodextrin	8	55 or less	30	Chloride
AllSport® Pepsico	Lemon-lime, fruit punch, orange, grape	High fructose corn syrup	8	55	55	Chloride, phosphorus, calcium
10–K® Suntory Water Group, Inc.	Lemon-lime, orange, fruit punch, lemonade, iced tea, pink lemonade, apple	Sucrose, glucose, fructose	6	55	30	Vitamin C, chloride, phosphorus
Quickick® Quick Kick	Lemon-lime, orange, fruit punch	High fructose corn syrup	7	100	23	Calcium, chloride, phosphorus
Endura® Meta Genics, Inc.	Orange, lemon-lime	Glucose polymers, fructose	6	46	80	Calcium, chloride, magnesium, chromium
1st Ade® American Beverages	Lemon-lime, orange, fruit punch	High fructose corn syrup, fructose	7	55	25	Phosphorus

TABLE 9-3
Fluid Replacement Beverages (continued)

BEVERAGE	FLAVORS	CARBOHYDRATE INGREDIENT	CARBOHYDRATE %(CONCENTRATION) PER 8 OZ	SODIUM (MG) PER 8 OZ	POTASSIUM (MG)	OTHER MINERALS AND VITAMINS
Hydra Fuel® Twin Labs	Orange, fruit punch, lemon-lime	Glucose polymers, glucose, fructose	7	25	50	Chloride, magnesium, chromium, phosphorus, vitamin C
Cytomax® Champion Nutrition	Fresh apple, tropical fruit, cool citrus	Corn starch, fructose, glucose	5	53	100	Chromium, magnesium
Gookinaid® Gookinaid ERG	Lemon, fruit punch, orange	Glucose	12	70	70	Vitamins A and C, calcium, iron
Pro Motion® Sports Beverage	Lemon-lime, fruit punch, orange, citrus cooler	Fructose	7.7	8	99	none
Everlast Sports Drink® A & W Beverages, Inc.	Lemon-lime, orange, mixed berry, grape	Sucrose, fructose	6	100	20	Vitamin C
PurePower® Energy & Recovery Drink Purepower Sports Nutrition	Lemon-lime, apple, tropical fruit	Fructose, maltodextrin	4.3	50	100	Chromium, vitamin C, calcium, phosphorus, magnesium
Breakthrough® Weider Health & Fitness	Lemon, tangerine, fruit punch, grape	Maltodextrin, fructose	8.5	60	45	Vitamin C, calcium, chloride, magnesium, riboflavin, niacin, iron, thiamin
Coca-Cola®	Regular, cherry	High fructose corn syrup, sucrose	11	6	Trace	Phosphorus

TABLE 9-3
Fluid-Replacement Beverages (continued)

BEVERAGE	FLAVORS	CARBOHYDRATE INGREDIENT	CARBOHYDRATE %(CONCENTRATION) PER 8 OZ	SODIUM (MG) PER 8 OZ	POTASSIUM (MG)	OTHER MINERALS AND VITAMINS
Diet soft drinks	All	None	0	2–8	18–100	Low phosphorous
Orange juice	—	Fructose, sucrose	10	6	436	Vitamins A and C, niacin, thiamin, riboflavin
Water	0	0	0	Low	Low	Low

The ideal fluid-replacement beverage for the athlete is rapidly absorbed, tastes good, and does not cause gastrointestinal problems when consumed in large volumes. Beyond these concerns, it's a matter of personal preference. You should try several different sports drinks during training to find the one that works the best.

ELECTROLYTES

Electrolytes such as sodium, chloride, and potassium are necessary for the maintenance of body fluid levels, muscle contraction, and nerve impulse transmission.

Sweating causes electrolyte losses (particularly sodium) as well as water losses. However, water losses during sweating are proportionately greater than electrolyte losses, so the body's cells actually end up with a greater electrolyte concentration.

The athlete's electrolyte needs can generally be met by consuming a balanced diet. Although sodium is the major electrolyte lost in sweat, our diets provide an abundance of salt (sodium chloride). The loss of 1 gram of sodium, which occurs with a 2-pound sweat loss, can easily be replaced by moderate salting of food. One-half teaspoon of salt supplies 1 gram of sodium.

Salt tablets should be avoided entirely. They can cause nausea due to irritation of the stomach lining, and they increase the body's water requirement.

Replacing potassium losses should not be a problem either. Athletes lose far more sodium than potassium during exercise. Orange juice, bananas, and potatoes are all excellent sources of potassium. Potassium supplements are unnecessary and can be dangerous. They can cause an excessively high level of potassium in the blood, resulting in an abnormal heart rhythm.

Electrolyte deficits, particularly sodium, can occur under certain conditions: when acclimating to a hot environment, following repeated workouts in hot weather, and during ultra-endurance events such as 50-mile runs, 100-mile bicycle rides, and long triathlons (such as the Ironman). Consuming only plain water during ultra-endurance events can cause a dangerous condition called hyponatremia (low blood sodium). Sodium losses in sweat during ultra-endurance events can be significant, and drinking only water dilutes the amount of sodium left in the blood.

Symptoms of low blood sodium include lethargy, muscle cramping, mental confusion, and seizures. Fortunately, this condition is rare—heat illnesses occur far more often. Hyponatremia can be prevented by consuming sports drinks that contain sodium.

Because sports drinks contain less sodium than found in sweat, consuming them can't cause a sodium overload. In addition to aiding fluid absorption during exercise, the sodium in sports drinks encourages fluid intake because it makes the drink taste better. Consuming sports drinks following exercise can also enhance rehydration. The sodium in the drink enables the athlete to retain water without inhibiting thirst.

ALCOHOL AND CAFFEINE

Drinking too much alcohol before exercise (even the night before) can harm performance. Alcohol is a diuretic that causes increased urination and water loss. The dehydrating effect of alcohol impairs performance and increases the risk of heat illnesses during exercise in warm weather.

Alcohol is a central nervous system depressant that reduces gross motor skills such as balance and coordination. It is metabolized by the liver, which can get rid of only about a half-ounce of alcohol per hour. Drinking alcohol before exercise decreases the output of glucose by the liver, thereby causing low blood glucose levels and early fatigue. Consuming alcohol during exercise in cold weather may also contribute to hypothermia (dangerously low body temperature).

Alcohol is a concentrated source of calories but does not contribute to the formation of muscle glycogen, the primary fuel for exercise. One 12-ounce beer or 5-ounce glass of wine supplies only 50 calories of carbohydrate—enough to run a half-mile. At the same time, these drinks supply one-half ounce of pure alcohol—a detrimental chemical responsible for traffic accidents and health problems.

Twelve ounces of beer, 5 ounces of wine, and 1½ ounces of hard liquor contain about equal quantities of alcohol. One or two drinks of this size daily appear to cause no harm to nonpregnant, healthy adult athletes who can afford the calories. Pregnant women should not drink since consumption of alcohol may cause birth defects or other problems during pregnancy.

Alcoholic beverages are high in calories and low in nutrients—a source of empty calories for adult athletes who wish to reduce their body fat. Athletes who drink should substitute alcohol calories for fat calories—not food calories. One 12-ounce beer provides 150 calories. A 5-ounce glass of wine or 1½ ounces of liquor each supply about 100 calories. Table 9-4 lists some common alcoholic beverages.

The caffeine found in coffee, tea, and some sodas is also a diuretic. Athletes who consume caffeinated beverages need to

TABLE 9-4
Alcoholic Beverages

BEVERAGE (% ALCOHOL BY VOLUME)	SERVING SIZE (OZ)	CALORIES
Wine (11.5%)	*5*	*105*
Sherry (19%)	*3*	*125*
Beer (4.5%)	*12*	*150*
Stout or porter on tap (about 3%)	*12*	*200*
Gin, vodka, rum, whiskey (rye, Scotch), 80 proof (40%)	*1.5*	*100–110*
Cordials, liqueurs, 25–100 proof (12.5–50%)	*1*	*50–100*
Martini (38%, 3/4 oz alcohol)	*2.5*	*156*
Manhattan (37%)	*2*	*128*
Bloody mary (12%)	*5*	*116*
Tom Collins (9%)	*7.5*	*121*
Daiquiri (28%)	*2*	*111*
Gin and tonic (9%)	*7.5*	*171*
Pina colada (12%)	*4.5*	*262*
Screwdriver (8%)	*7*	*174*
Tequila sunrise (14%)	*5.5*	*189*
Whiskey sour prepared from bottled mix (17%)	*3.5*	*160*

pay extra attention to their fluid intake at rest and during exercise. Diet caffeinated sodas, which are frequently chosen by weight-conscious athletes, are especially poor rehydration beverages due to increased urine production.

10

BODY COMPOSITION

IN OUR SOCIETY, THE BATHROOM SCALE has a following worthy of a political party or religion. An unbelievable number of weight-loss gimmicks have been spawned by our obsession with weight loss. In the rush to shed pounds, a very important question is often overlooked: "How fat am I?"

The scale cannot differentiate between fat pounds and muscle pounds. The scale does not indicate how fat a person is, because both fat and muscle, as well as bone and water, contribute to the total weight.

The term "overweight" refers only to body weight in excess of the average for a specific height. The term "underweight" refers only to the body weight below the average weight for height. The scale is biased against stocky, muscular people, just as it favors thin, slightly built people.

A more accurate indicator of fitness is body composition, which divides weight into two categories. One is the fat-free mass, of which muscle is a major component. The other category is fat. What is really important is how much of an athlete's weight is fat. This is expressed as *percent body fat*.

It is now recognized that weight alone is not a suitable indicator of performance capability. This means that an athlete's "goal weight range" shouldn't be based on the individual's existing scale weight. Instead, the athlete should have her or his body composition assessed, in which the amounts of lean and fat tissue are evaluated.

Many athletes ask what weight, or range of weights, will help them achieve optimal performance. It's true that extra weight can harm performance, particularly when the body must be moved through space, as in running or jumping. Although some weight loss may improve performance, too much can impair performance and jeopardize the athlete's health.

The person who suffers the most when evaluated by weight alone is the stocky, muscular woman or man. Because these athletes may have little fat, they weigh more than average because of a large fat-free mass. To lose weight, they may lose muscle and experience a deterioration in their performance. This is just one reason why it is so important to have body composition assessed before trying to lose weight.

Athletes are somewhat restricted by their genetic inheritance. Body shape and size are largely determined by skeleton size, since a certain amount of muscle and tissue accompany a certain amount of bone. Beyond heredity, the total amount and distribution of muscle mass will depend on the type of training you do. For example, weight training increases muscle mass more than running.

As athletes know, body type is important in most sports, and each sport seems to require a certain body type. The large, muscular person will never be an elite marathoner, just as an elite marathoner would not survive as an interior lineman on the football field.

Whereas body size and shape can be altered only slightly, substantial changes can occur in body composition. These changes can significantly affect your performance. In power sports, performance can be improved by extra muscle gained from weight lifting. It is also obvious that some sports can be harmed by excess body fat. However, athletes who train for a specific sport are likely to have the muscle mass that is appropriate for that sport. If, because of genetics, their muscle mass is greater than desired, they will only hurt themselves by trying to lose weight.

BODY FAT STANDARDS

Many athletes ask what percent body fat they should have to achieve peak performance. While numerous studies have been done on athletes, the results suggest that body fat values differ widely both between sports and within sports. Thus, an ideal body fat for a particular sport is difficult to establish. Table 10-1 shows the ranges of relative body fat for men and women in various sports.

Before attempting to achieve a certain percent body fat, there are several things to keep in mind. An athlete's success in a sport depends on a variety of factors. Having a low body fat does not, in itself, ensure that the person will be an elite athlete.

The target percentage of body fat for men for general health is around 15%. A desirable level of body fat for women for general health is around 22%. Three percent of the total body fat in men is considered "essential fat." It appears that a man cannot reduce his body fat below this limit without impairing his physiological function and capacity for exercise.

The percentage of body fat considered "essential" for women is 12%. This higher level of fat is related to child-bearing functions and takes into account sex-specific fat in the breasts, hips, and other tissues.

As an upper limit, athletes should try to be close to the generally desirable body fat levels of 15% for men and 22% for women. Otherwise, an athlete's ideal percent body fat is where he/she performs the best. Attempting to reach an unrealistic percent body fat can set athletes back as much as attempting to reach an unrealistic weight.

In general, weight and percent body fat should be monitored by a health professional and titrated down to a level where

TABLE 10-1
Ranges of Relative Body Fat
for Men and Women Athletes in Various Sports

SPORT	MEN	WOMEN
Baseball, softball	8–14	12–18
Basketball	6–12	10–16
Body building	5–8	6–12
Canoeing and kayaking	6–12	10–16
Cycling	5–11	8–15
Fencing	8–12	10–16
Football	6–18	—
Golf	10–16	12–20
Gymnastics	5–12	8–16
Horse racing	6–12	10–16
Ice and field hockey	8–16	12–18
Orienteering	5–12	8–16
Pentathlon	—	8–15
Racketball	6–14	10–18
Rowing	6–14	8–16
Rugby	6–16	—
Skating	5–12	8–16
Skiing	7–15	10–18
Ski jumping	7–15	10–18
Soccer	6–14	10–18
Swimming	6–12	10–18
Synchronized swimming	—	10–18
Tennis	6–14	10–20
Track and field		
Running events	5–12	8–15
Field events	8–18	12–20
Triathlon	5–12	8–15
Volleyball	7–15	10–18
Weight lifting	5–12	10–18
Wrestling	5–16	—

■ **Source:** Adapted from J. H. Wilmore and D. L. Costill, *Physiology of Sport and Exercise* (Champaign; IL: Human Kinetics, 1994).

performance is optimal. For one female athlete, that may be 110 pounds and 15% body fat, for another female athlete it may be 160 pounds and 22% body fat.

HYDROSTATIC WEIGHING

The hydrostatic (underwater) weighing procedure involves weighing the athlete on a balance beam scale and then determining the weight of the athlete submerged under water. Because muscle is denser than fat (1 lb of muscle takes up the room of ⅓ lb of fat), athletes with more muscle and less fat will weigh more underwater. In other words, they will have a higher body density and lower percent body fat.

Hydrostatic weighing utilizes Archimedes' principle for assessing body volume. Archimedes discovered that the volume of an object can be determined by its loss of weight in water (that is, its actual weight minus its weight under water).

Knowing the volume of a body and its mass or weight makes it possible to calculate density. The density of the body is then determined through a simple formula:

$$\text{Density} = \text{Weight/Volume}$$

Once the body density has been assessed from hydrostatic weighing, percentage body fat can be estimated.

Even though there are certain technical limitations to this procedure, underwater weighing has been referred to as the "gold standard," because it is the most accurate technique currently available to assess body composition. Underwater weighing is shown in Figure 10-1.

ANTHROPOMETRY MEASUREMENTS OF BODY COMPOSITION

Anthropometry is generally divided into the measurements of skinfold thicknesses, circumferences, and bone diameters. Measurements

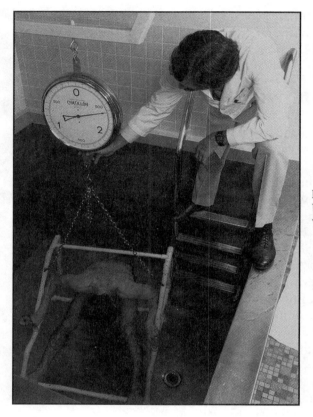

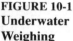

**FIGURE 10-1
Underwater
Weighing**

from different anatomical sites are used in mathematical equations
to predict body density and percent body fat. These prediction
equations have been validated against other criterion methods,
typically the "gold standard" of underwater weighing.

Like most clinical techniques of measuring body composition, anthropometry is indirect, which increases the measurement
error. Just as with underwater weighing, percent body fat results
obtained by anthropometry should be considered *estimates*—
never absolute values. Brief descriptions are provided below for
skinfold measures, circumferences, and bone diameters.

Skinfolds are the best method to use if underwater weighing
is not available or practical. As shown in Figure 10-2, skinfold

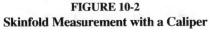

FIGURE 10-2
Skinfold Measurement with a Caliper

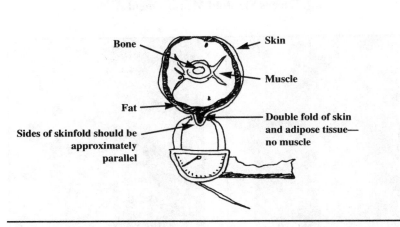

measurements represent the thickness of a double layer of skin and the underlying subcutaneous fat, as determined by metal (not plastic) calipers. The usefulness of skinfold measures is threefold. First, measurements are used for estimating percentage body fat. Second, skinfold thickness is used in determining regional distribution of subcutaneous fat. Last, using skinfolds with circumferences can help to estimate muscle and bone changes.

Although procedures for taking skinfold measures are straightforward, the examiner must be properly trained in the specific anatomic skinfold sites (e.g., triceps, thigh, abdomen) and have had sufficient practice to take consistent measurements. Which skinfold sites are selected is based on the purpose of the measurement and the mathematical prediction equation chosen. Figure 10-3 illustrates a triceps skinfold measurement.

Even in trained hands, the error in predicting percent body fat with skinfolds is 3%, on average. This means that an athlete whose body fat is estimated to be 15% could be as low as 12%

FIGURE 10-3
Triceps Skinfold Measurement

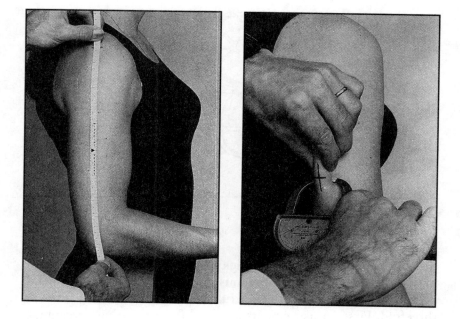

or as high as 18%. This is why it is best to provide a range of desirable body fat values for an athlete.

Circumference, or girth, measures are affected by skin, muscle, fat, and bone. Circumference measures, when used alone or in combination with skinfold measures, help to evaluate fat patterning, muscular development, and frame size. Measurements appear easy to make, but obtaining accurate measures can be challenging. Measures are taken with a plastic or metal tape measure at specific body sites such as the chest, waist, hip, upper arm, or thigh, as shown in Figure 10-4.

The measurement of *bone breadth* (joint width) is used to assess frame size and skeletal mass. Body weight varies with bone thickness, as well as with height and age. An individual with a greater bone weight has a greater body weight. Knowing

FIGURE 10-4
Measurement of Chest Circumference

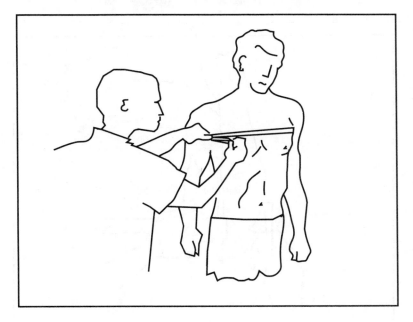

frame size helps to distinguish those who are overweight due to a large fat-free mass (bone and muscle) and those whose extra weight is predominantly fat.

Bone breadth is measured with broad-blade anthropometers and small sliding calipers. Common sites selected for an estimation of frame size and skeletal mass are the elbow and the wrist, as shown in Figure 10-5.

OTHER METHODS OF MEASURING BODY COMPOSITION

Bioelectrical impedance (BIA) is a technique that involves passing a small electrical current throughout the body and measuring

FIGURE 10-5
Elbow Breadth Measurement at the Epicondyles of the Humerus

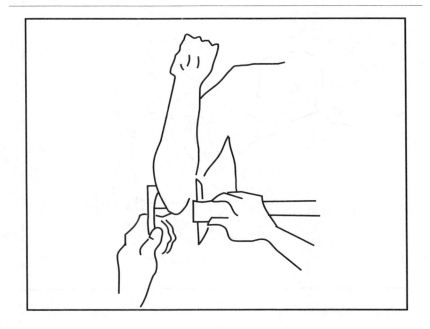

the resistance encountered (through electrodes placed on the hands and feet). This method is based on the fact that lean tissue is a good conductor of electricity, whereas fat is not. BIA is essentially a measure of total body water, which is used to estimate lean body mass. Fat weight is then calculated by subtracting lean body weight from body weight.

BIA has become popularized (especially in health clubs) because it's an easy, quick, noninvasive technique. Unfortunately, BIA tends to overestimate the body fat of a lean person and underestimate the body fat of an obese person. The method assumes that the athlete is completely hydrated when the measure is taken. Results must be viewed with caution, as considerable error is possible.

The *infrared interactance* technique uses a fiber-optic probe that is pressed against the skin. A light beam is emitted that penetrates the subcutaneous fat and muscle and is reflected off the bone to a silicon detector in the probe. The procedure takes only 2 to 3 minutes to complete, and the subject is fully clothed.

This procedure involves only one measurement site: the biceps muscles on the arm. Percent fat is estimated from a mathematical equation that incorporates the probe's optical density measurement with the individual's age, weight, height, and exercise level. This procedure is only in the early stages of development, and the validity of using a single site to represent the total body must be questioned.

A number of other laboratory-based techniques are also available for the assessment of body composition. Some are primarily experimental, so their potential for screening of athletes or for testing of the general public is either limited or unknown. Some of the techniques that you may have heard of are magnetic resonance imaging (MRI), spectrometry, radiography, dual-photon absorptiometry, and total body electrical conductivity (TOBEC). Of these methods, dual-photon absorptiometry, in which the bone mineral content and soft tissue content of the body are determined, has recently been shown to have considerable promise for the evaluation of body composition.

SPECIAL CONSIDERATIONS FOR EVALUATING CHILDREN AND YOUTH

Evaluation in children and youth is complicated by several factors that affect the conceptual basis for estimating fat and lean tissue. Compared to adults, children have higher body water content and lower bone mineral content. This means their body density is lower than that of adults. Mathematical equations used for adults are not appropriate for children because they may overestimate body fat by 3–6% and underestimate lean tissue.

Another limitation is that the chemical composition of the fat-free mass changes as the child passes through puberty. Estimates of body fat by skinfolds, bone diameters, and circumferences may reflect alterations in the composition of the fat-free body components, which include water, mineral, and protein, rather than alterations in actual fat content. Because of this, special mathematical equations have been developed that are appropriate to use when evaluating body composition in children and adolescents.

Lastly, the body composition tables that show percent body fat values for male and female athletes are not suitable for children because most of these measurements were taken on older athletes. There are currently no standards of comparison for young athletes that are specific for sport and gender. Just as with adult athletes, no tables are available that provide an "optimal or ideal weight" for performance (if one does in fact exist).

INAPPROPRIATE USE OF WEIGHT/BODY FAT STANDARDS

From a practical standpoint, body composition measures can be used by a qualified health professional to monitor changes in fat and lean tissue during training. When used inappropriately, the results can be disastrous, and the athlete is driven to lose more weight to achieve a certain percentage of body fat. The athlete is likely to experience declines in performance and health when her or his weight drops below a certain level.

Numerous factors contribute to this deterioration, depending on the sport and the particular athlete. Extreme weight loss can disrupt nutritional status, hormone levels, bone mineral density, psychological functioning, and (for young athletes) growth rate.

Chronic fatigue often accompanies major weight loss. The sources of this fatigue have not been clearly identified, but both the central nervous system and the hormonal (endocrine) system appear to be involved. Depleted fuel stores probably play a role. When athletes train hard and consume a diet that is inadequate in total calories or carbohydrate calories, liver and muscle glycogen stores become depleted. This depletion of the body's carbohydrate stores causes weakness, fatigue, and impaired performance.

When the body is forced to use protein for fuel, significant losses of muscle protein occur, which can lead to fatigue. Inadequate intake of calories, vitamins, and minerals have been reported for many different athletes who focus on low body weight during training.

Although body composition measurements are helpful in evaluating the fitness and performance of mature athletes, they should *never* be used in the prepubescent athlete to manipulate body fat for sports participation or to set stringent weight-loss guidelines. Doing so may harm the child athlete's growth and development.

THE ATHLETIC FEMALE TRIAD

There is increasing evidence that disordered eating (anorexia), menstrual dysfunction (amenorrhea), and bone mineral disorders (reduced bone mineral density and increased risk of fractures) form a triad of disorders in certain female athletes.

Constant focus on either achieving or maintaining a prescribed goal weight, particularly if unreasonable, may lead to disordered eating or a full-blown eating disorder. A high prevalence of scanty (oligomenorrhea) or absent menstruation (amenorrhea) and delayed onset of menstruation (menarche) have also been associated with low-body-weight or low-body-fat sports. There is a direct relationship between menstrual dysfunction (low estrogen levels) and low bone mineral density. This increases the risk of stress fractures and early osteoporosis (see Chapter 13).

Although bone mineral density does increase with the resumption of normal menses, it appears that the regain of bone is limited so that bone density remains significantly below normal levels even when menstrual function returns to normal.

11

WEIGHT CONTROL: LOSING FAT

WEIGHT LOSS, WEIGHT MAINTENANCE, OR WEIGHT GAIN is a matter of energy balance. Your body weight will stay the same when your calorie intake equals your calorie expenditure. To lose weight, energy expenditure must be greater than energy intake; whereas to gain weight, energy intake must be greater than energy expenditure. If you want to lose weight, you must eat less, exercise more, or do both.

Everyone has a specific requirement for calories. Age, gender, weight, and physical activity determine your caloric needs. The caloric cost of the sport depends on the frequency, intensity, and duration of the activity. The more intense the exercise and the longer it's carried out, the greater the caloric cost. Sedentary individuals require about 30 calories per kilogram daily (14 calories per pound), whereas active athletes require 50 calories per kilogram daily (23 calories per pound) or more.

DIET AND WEIGHT-LOSS

The American College of Sports Medicine has provided guidelines for desirable weight-loss programs. Adults should consume at least 1,200 calories to meet nutritional needs. The daily caloric deficit can range from 500 to 1,000 calories, depending on the person's caloric requirement. The rate of sustained weight loss should not exceed 2 pounds per week (1 pound of fat equals 3,500 calories). This mild caloric restriction results in a manageable loss of fat and minimizes loss of water, electrolytes, minerals, and lean body mass.

Caloric intake can be reduced by eating fewer empty calories—foods high in sugar, fat, and alcohol. Eating habits can also be improved by eating more slowly and avoiding seconds. The meal frequency of the diet is also important. Skipping meals earlier in the day is more likely to cause overeating in the evening, so structured meal patterns around training and competition can facilitate weight control.

The low-fat, high-complex carbohydrate diet recommended by the U.S. Dietary Guidelines promotes fat loss for several reasons. Since fat is a concentrated source of calories, reducing fat intake will automatically reduce caloric intake. Dietary fat is also more fattening than dietary carbohydrate because dietary fat is more likely to be stored as body fat. The conversion of dietary carbohydrate to body fat is metabolically costly: About 23% of the carbohydrate calories are expended in the energy conversion process. The conversion of dietary fat to body fat is easy and requires little energy: About 3% of the fat calories are expended in the conversion process.

Athletes will perform at their best if they reduce to their best competitive weight (while adequately hydrated) either in the off-season or early in the competitive season. Allowing for increases in lean tissue and a reduction of body fat as a result of training, the athlete should maintain that weight throughout the season.

EXERCISE AND BODY FAT LOSS

An effective weight-loss regimen incorporates aerobic exercise and resistance training. Athletes who don't expend many calories in their sport (e.g., gymnastics, baseball) can benefit by adding an aerobic exercise program to increase their caloric expenditure.

Though the goal of an exercise program is to reduce fat tissue while preserving lean tissue, using caloric restriction alone leads to significant losses of lean (muscle) tissue. A reduction in muscle mass can significantly reduce caloric needs. In fact, caloric restriction can reduce the resting metabolic rate, and so lower caloric expenditure, by as much as 15%.

Aerobic exercise promotes body fat loss more than resistance training due to the greater caloric expenditure. However, resistance training increases lean weight more than aerobic exercise. By increasing the proportion of lean tissue to body fat, both exercises increase the body's calorie-burning ability, since lean weight requires more calories for maintenance than body fat. In fact, metabolic rate is closely tied to muscle mass—the greater the muscle mass, the greater the caloric requirement. These changes in body composition, along with the actual energy cost of exercising, significantly increase the body's caloric needs.

An exercise session can also increase the resting metabolic rate and so increase caloric requirements slightly. The metabolic rate may remain elevated after moderate exercise (60% of $\dot{V}O_{2max}$ or about 70% of maximal heart rate) lasting 40 minutes or longer. The added calories equal about 5–6% of the total caloric cost of the activity. Although small, this increased caloric expenditure, over and above the energy cost of the exercise itself, can aid weight loss over a period of time.

Combining exercise with caloric restriction reduces the loss of lean tissue experienced with caloric restriction. Combining diet and exercise also promotes faster body fat loss than when either is used alone.

The individual desiring body fat loss should include aerobic exercise 3 to 5 days per week, for 30 to 60 minutes, at 60–90% of maximal heart rate (50–85% $\dot{V}O_{2max}$). Increased exercise frequency and duration (5 days a week for 60 minutes) are associated with greater fat loss due to increased caloric expenditure. The exercise intensity should be lower for an individual with a low initial level of fitness.

The goal is to expend 300 calories per exercise session for a total weekly caloric expenditure of at least 1,000 calories, since this seems to represent a threshold for body fat loss. In practical terms, 300 calories is roughly equal to walking or jogging 3 miles, swimming 1 mile, or bicycling 12 miles, or an aerobics class (including warm-up and cool-down). If the intensity of the exercise is low, the person exercises longer to burn off the calories. A low-intensity workout that burns off 300 calories in an hour is just as beneficial for weight control as a high-intensity workout that burns off 300 calories in 30 minutes.

Exercise draws from all the fat stores of the body. Some exercises improve muscle tone in specific areas and make the person look thinner, which is a desirable outcome. Sit-ups, for example, tone the abdomen and so reduce abdominal girth, but they don't burn off the "tummy roll."

UNHEALTHY WEIGHT-LOSS METHODS

Gradual weight loss through sound nutrition and exercise strategies are the best plan for fat loss. Unfortunately, many people resort to unhealthy weight-loss techniques to shed pounds rapidly such as fad diets, fasting, severe caloric restriction, diet pills, and fluid restriction. As a result, both health and performance are compromised.

Fad diets are typically low in carbohydrate and cause muscle and liver glycogen depletion. Since water is stored with glycogen, a large amount of water is lost. The individual may erroneously attribute this weight loss to a reduction in fat stores. However, fat stores are virtually untouched—instead, the person is dehydrated. Complications of low-carbohydrate diets include ketosis (increased blood acids from fat breakdown), hypoglycemia (low blood sugar), potassium and calcium depletion, weakness, nausea, and electrolyte loss. Inadequate intake of protein, vitamins, and minerals is also a concern on such unbalanced regimens.

Fasting, semistarvation, and fluid-restricted diets are dangerous for the athlete. Lack of important nutrients aside, fatigue, dehydration, electrolyte imbalances, and loss of muscle, liver glycogen, and lean tissue can occur. For the still-growing child athlete, the risks are even greater.

These weight-loss regimens are also inappropriate from a behavioral standpoint, because they tend to reinforce faulty eating habits and do not result in healthy long-term weight control. People who lose weight this way usually regain the weight they lost and may end up even heavier than when they started.

Diet pills should never be self-prescribed. They typically contain a stimulant such as amphetamines to suppress appetite. However, this appetite-suppressant effect is temporary and weight loss decreases with time. Amphetamines can be addictive and cause insomnia, high blood pressure, headaches, and dizziness. Phenylpropanolamine, another hunger-controlling ingredient, has been shown to cause high blood pressure, irregular heart rhythm, and liver damage.

Rubber or plastic suits or heavy clothing worn during exercise in an effort to "melt away" fat are dangerous and ineffective. Again, weight loss is from fluid loss, not fat reduction. This strategy prevents the evaporation of perspiration, which is crucial to temperature regulation. Dehydration, heat illness, and even heatstroke may be the result. Saunas also cause water loss, which is only temporary and quickly replaced when the person quenches her thirst.

SPOT REDUCTION

Spot reduction to eliminate so-called cellulite from specific areas of the body is also vigorously promoted by creators of creams, pills and "special" exercise equipment. The reality is that cellulite is simply subcutaneous fat that has a dimpled appearance. The only way to get rid of fat deposits is through diet and exercise. There is no way any cream, massage, or exercise can reduce fat on one part of the body.

Vibrating and elastic belts are completely ineffective. The claim that they "break up" fat has no basis in fact. Although the vibration may relax the person and improve his general feeling of well-being, such passive exercise does not increase a person's caloric expenditure and cannot decrease body fat. Similarly, elastic belts cannot "melt away" fat. They may cause temporary water loss from the area or compress the tissues so that the waistline looks thinner for a short time.

Electric muscle stimulators, placed on specific muscle groups, discharge a small electric current, causing the muscles to contract. These devices have no effect on fat deposits, though they may help soothe or rehabilitate injured muscles.

EVALUATING WEIGHT-LOSS PROGRAMS

All of these gimmicks do not address the problems of eating habits, lifestyle, and metabolism, and so cannot be recommended for weight loss. When evaluating a weight-loss program, you should consider the following points:

1. Does the diet include a variety of foods to ensure nutritional adequacy? Be wary of diets that eliminate certain foods entirely or promote eating them in "special fat-burning combinations."
2. Does the program avoid sensational claims such as magic, "quick and easy," "metabolically proven," "eat all you want and still lose weight," "burns fat and builds muscle," and "energizing"?
3. Is the diet's effectiveness well documented by research published in credible scientific journals (consult a registered dietitian) and not based on testimonials by famous people or self-proclaimed experts?
4. Does it include modification of eating patterns and exercise?
5. Does it avoid the use of diuretics and/or appetite suppressants?
6. Does it consider the special needs of athletes (fluids, calories, carbohydrates, etc.)? Weight-loss patterns of athletes may be influenced by many factors, including intensity, frequency and duration of training, stipulations of coach or parents, personal goals, misconceptions about nutrition and body composition, and the inherent demands of the sport (frequency of competition and length of the competitive season).

ENERGY EFFICIENCY

A low body weight and/or percentage of body fat provides a competitive edge or is aesthetically important for sports such as distance running, gymnastics, figure skating, ballet, and diving. Other sports, such as wrestling, impose specific weight limits for competition. This means that some athletes keep their weight continually low, some lose weight during the competitive season and gain it in the off-season, and others lose weight periodically throughout the competitive season (e.g., wrestlers who need to "make weight").

Low caloric intakes have been reported for many of these athletes, which is not surprising since low body weight is a focus of training. However, some athletes are not even consuming the RDA for calories for their age and gender. This is striking considering that the activity level of the sport is not considered in the RDA. Do these athletes really need fewer calories?

One theory is that these athletes have become energy efficient so that their bodies have adapted to fewer calories. However, it's also possible that the lower caloric intakes observed in "energy efficient" athletes are due to underreporting of the amount of food eaten. At the present, it isn't clear whether or not "energy efficiency" exists among low-body-weight athletes.

FOCUS ON BODY COMPOSITION

Body weight usually changes very little, if any, in the first few weeks of an exercise program. This is because lean (muscle) weight initially increases at about the same rate that fat weight is being lost. Individuals can become discouraged, because the scales show no change, even though body composition (fat versus lean) is changing dramatically. During this time, the person should pay more attention to how clothing fits than what the scale says.

It is even possible to gain weight while losing fat (particularly when including resistance training) because of correspondingly greater muscle gain. For example, a person can gain four pounds of muscle but lose two pounds of fat. This often happens to sedentary women who begin exercising. They may drop two dress sizes but gain two pounds. Some have even quit exercising when this happens because they're conditioned to go by scale weight.

It's a good idea to have body composition evaluated before trying to lose or gain weight, and again periodically to measure any muscle gain and fat loss from exercise. Scale weight isn't an accurate indicator of body composition, and does not give people the real picture of the changes expected from regular exercise.

12

SPECIAL CASES:
GAINING MUSCLE, "MAKING WEIGHT," AND WORKING WITH OVERWEIGHT ACTIVE CHILDREN

ATHLETES WHO RECEIVE GUIDELINES on weight control, nutrition, and fitness are less likely to develop health and body weight problems. Once they recognize that a certain percentage of body fat is healthy and even required for optimal performance, athletes may resist the temptation of becoming thin at all costs. With the guidance from health professionals and support from family and coaches, the athlete can achieve a healthy competitive weight through training and a balanced diet that meets nutrient needs and caloric requirements for weight loss or weight gain.

GAINING MUSCLE

Many athletes have as much difficulty gaining weight as the average person has losing weight. Athletes may want to gain weight for several reasons. Increased muscle mass can aid performance in strength and power sports. Body builders gain weight for aesthetic purposes.

Ideally, the weight gained should be muscle rather than fat so that the new tissue can be used to produce force. Thus, the ideal weight-gain program combines progressive resistance exercise (weight training) at least three times a week with increased caloric intake.

A reasonable amount of lean weight that can be gained weekly is about one pound. To gain 1 pound a week, the athlete must increase caloric intake by 350 calories per day (a pound of muscle contains about 2,500 calories). In addition, the caloric cost of weight training (about 200 calories per hour workout) must be added. These calories are above and beyond the amount the athlete normally requires to maintain body weight in his or her sport.

The program to gain weight should begin with the athlete keeping at least a three-day diet record. This will give a good indication of how much is being eaten to maintain present weight and how much more needs to be consumed to gain weight.

The athlete can start to increase caloric intake by eating larger servings of the foods currently being eaten (just the opposite of what would be recommended for a weight-loss program). Meal patterns can be adjusted to incorporate additional calories by adding mid-morning, mid-afternoon, and bedtime snacks. Alternatively, five or six small meals can be eaten throughout the day. The athlete can drink commercial or homemade liquid meals with regular meals or as a snack.

For example, a person requiring 2,000 calories per day wants to gain weight. She needs an additional 2,500 calories to gain 1 pound of muscle. She also requires 200 calories per session of weight training, which is done five times per week for a total of 1,000 calories per week. When the extra calories for muscle gain and increased training are added, the person needs to consume an additional 3,500 calories per week, or 500 extra calories per day. This raises the overall caloric requirement to 2,500 calories per day.

Bulky, low-calorie foods such as cereals, grains, and salads should be discouraged. They are too filling in relation to the amount of calories they provide.

Fats have a high caloric density and so help to increase an athlete's food intake. However, fats should not provide more than 30% of caloric intake, with emphasis on unsaturated and monounsaturated fats, due to the adverse health effects of high dietary percentages of saturated fats.

Many athletes consume a high-protein diet and/or take protein and amino acid supplements to gain weight. The research on protein requirements during training suggests that athletes need to consume at least 1.2 gm per kg of body weight daily and may benefit from up to 1.7 gm per kg during periods of muscle building. This amount can be easily met with diet, so athletes do not need protein supplements.

Protein consumption in athletes is much greater when their caloric intake increases as a result of training. A diet supplying 12–15% of the calories from protein is adequate to increase muscle mass. To gain 1 pound of muscle a week represents an additional 14 grams of protein, which is easily supplied by 1 cup of nonfat milk and 1 ounce of chicken (15 grams total).

When supplements or the diet supplies more amino acids than can be incorporated into new proteins, the excess amino acids are either burned for energy or converted to fat. Either way, the result is excess urea production, which increases the body's water requirement since extra water is necessary to help excrete the extra urea load.

If the athlete insists on taking a protein supplement, nonfat powered milk is a high-quality, inexpensive protein supplement (¼ cup provides 11 grams of protein) without the unproved additives that many "weight gainer" supplements contain.

As when losing weight, athletes wishing to gain weight need periodic body composition assessments to ensure they're gaining muscle and not fat. An increase in scale weight of more than one pound a week suggests fat gain or anabolic steroid usage.

Anabolic Steroids

Despite the fact that anabolic steroids are banned by the United States Olympic Committee, National Collegiate Athletic Association, and other sport-governing bodies, their use by athletes is widespread. Weight lifters, power lifters, and body builders appear to be the most frequent users of anabolic steroids. The percentage is slightly lower among track and field athletes (shot put, javelin, and discus) and football players. In general, steroid use is significantly less in females than in males.

Anabolic steroids are used by athletes for several reasons. The primary purpose is to improve performance by increasing muscle mass for strength or physique. Research has shown that anabolic steroids in combination with intensive weight training does increase muscle mass. For the endurance athlete, steroids have been of interest because they may help to stimulate red blood cell production. Although anabolic steroids may help to increase red blood cell production for certain types of anemia, steroids are not beneficial for people with normal red blood cell levels. Steroids don't increase maximal oxygen uptake or aerobic endurance. There is also no evidence to support the belief that steroids will facilitate recovery in athletes after intense training.

How do anabolic steroids work? Male hormones, principally testosterone, are partially responsible for the developmental changes that occur during puberty and adolescence. Male hormones exert both androgenic and anabolic effects. Androgenic effects include the development of primary and secondary sex characteristics such as facial hair, voice changes, maturation of the sex glands, and increased aggressiveness. Anabolic effects include growth and development of muscle and bone and enhanced neural conduction. Anabolic steroids have been manufactured to maximize the anabolic effects (tissue building) and minimize the androgenic effects (sex-linked). However, certain-undesirable side effects can still occur.

Anabolic steroids are available for use by oral consumption or injection. Table 12-1 lists some of the most commonly used anabolic steroids in the United States. Although the therapeutic dose varies for the different steroids, a normal level is about 5–10 mg/day for oral compounds. Athletes have been reported to use between 10 and 300 milligrams per day, with some reports being as high as 2,000 mg. Some athletes practice "stacking," which involves taking two or more steroids at one time.

TABLE 12-1
Trade and Generic Names of the Most Commonly Used
Anabolic Steroids in the United States

ORAL COMPOUNDS	INJECTABLE COMPOUNDS
Anadrol (oxymetholone)	*Deca-durabolin (nandrolone decanoate)*
Anavar (oxandrolone)	*Depo-testosterone (testosterone cypionate)*
Dianabol (methandienone)	*Durabolin (nandrolone phenylpropionate)*
Maxibolin (ethylestrenol)	*Primobolan-depot (methenolone enanthate)*
Winstrol (stanozolol)	

Although anabolic steroids increase muscle mass, they present serious health risks that could be life-threatening. Some of the reported physical symptoms include acne, baldness, fluid retention, oily skin, deepening of the voice, hair growth on face and body, breast enlargement in males, and reduced sperm production. For prepubescent children, steroid use can result in stunted growth. Personality changes range from mild aggressiveness to extreme hostility ("roid rage"). The most serious health problems associated with steroid use are liver damage and premature development of coronary heart disease. Anabolic steroids are also weak carcinogens and may increase the risk of cancer.

THE SPECIAL CASE OF WRESTLERS— "MAKING WEIGHT"

Scholastic wrestlers must meet a certain weight classification in order to compete. It is a common practice throughout the competitive season for wrestlers to restrict food and fluid intake in order to compete at one to three weight classes below their normal weight. Wrestlers typically believe that this practice, known as "making weight," gives them a competitive edge over smaller opponents. Few wrestlers, coaches, and parents realize the negative physiological impact this practice may have on the wrestlers' bodies.

Making weight lowers blood and plasma volumes, impairs heart function during submaximal work (e.g., higher heart rate, smaller stroke volume, and reduced cardiac output), harms body temperature control, decreases kidney blood flow and kidney filtration, and increases electrolyte losses. The caloric and micronutrient content of a wrestler's diet during training is typically inadequate.

From a performance standpoint, making weight can lead to liver and muscle glycogen depletion, dehydration, reduced muscular strength, and decreased performance work time. Since wrestlers rarely regain all of their lost weight after the official weigh-in prior to competition, they may be wrestling under suboptimal conditions.

All coaches, parents, and athletes must be alerted to the consequences of rapid and extreme weight reduction by fluid and food restriction and to the healthy alternatives for achieving a suitable competitive weight. In an effort to preclude the use of erratic weight-loss practices commonly observed among adolescent wrestlers, it is imperative to establish the following healthy weight-loss guidelines:

- *Estimate minimal wrestling weight.* This is the lowest weight class an athlete should compete at based on a fat level of 5–7%. This should be determined by body composition assessment shortly after school begins in the fall. Early determination of optimal weight allows sufficient time for gradual weight loss before the competitive season begins.
- *Re-evaluate minimal wrestling weight during the season to account for changes in weight due to growth.* Growth rates for adolescent males vary greatly—they can gain about 10 pounds per year, or approximately 3 pounds during the third of the year represented by the wrestling season. In most states, regulations allow for a weight gain of 1 to 2 pounds during each of the winter months to allow for normal maturation.
- *Encourage consultation with a sports nutritionist to address individual caloric and nutrient needs.* This is highly recommended, but not always feasible. At a minimum, athletes

should have a group lecture by a nutritionist and educational materials that address the essentials of nutrition (energy balance, tips for reducing fat in the diet while increasing nutrient density, pre- and postevent eating). The consequences of crash weight-reduction techniques on performance and the importance of hydration should be emphasized.

- *Wrestlers should consume at least 2,000 calories daily.* Although calorie needs vary among individual athletes, this amount promotes an appropriate weight loss (no more than 2 lb per week) while meeting nutrient needs for growth and intense training.

- *Include parents in the educational process.* This may entail providing strategies for parents on recipe modification, low-fat snack ideas, and low-calorie beverages for hydration. The dangers of "cutting weight" and appropriate methods of weight loss need to be made clear. The positive aspects of healthy weight control, and wrestling workouts that result in a more muscular and fit athlete, should be underscored.

- *Give special consideration to the football player who wants to participate in wrestling.* They typically compete at the upper weight classes and may end the football season with a higher than desirable amount of body fat and little time for weight reduction before wrestling season begins. These athletes should be identified during football season. Then, weight-loss efforts can be initiated earlier to enhance their performance in football and prepare them for wrestling. Aside from caloric reduction, often two aerobic training sessions are needed per week to facilitate fat loss. Weight loss in these heavier athletes should not be greater than 2 lbs per week.

- *Advocate slow, extended weight loss.* Repeated weight loss and regain (weight cycling) should be avoided as it may potentially have negative effects on nutrient intake, metabolism, performance, and health. However, too little is known about weight fluctuation in athletes to issue stern warnings about long-term health effects.

WORKING WITH THE OVERWEIGHT ACTIVE CHILD

Obesity (a weight that is 20% above healthy body weight) is an increasing problem among children and adolescents in the United States and occurs as a result of a complex interaction of genetic and environmental factors. Children are also becoming obese at younger ages, and obesity that occurs earlier and persists throughout childhood is more difficult to treat. Even though the health complications of obesity are fewer for children and adolescents than adults, obesity that continues into adulthood may lead to hypertension, diabetes, and heart disease. From a psychological standpoint, a major concern accompanying chronic childhood obesity is the potential for emotional upsets and loss of self-esteem that may be caused by the stigma of being overweight.

Although obesity is an important health problem and prevalence is increasing, efforts by coaches or parents to eliminate excess body fat by requiring the obese child to exercise excessively can be too sudden or too extreme. The obese child participating in sports needs a medically supervised weight-control program that focuses on weight monitoring, caloric reduction as described in Chapter 11, and gradual increased activity. Several strategies for working with the obese child during a weight-reduction plan are outlined below for coaches and parents.

Coaches

- Never single out the obese child by asking him or her to run extra laps or exercise longer than other children.
- Never restrict fluids for any child.
- Never refer to the child as being obese or chubby, especially in front of his or her teammates.
- Watch for signs of heat distress. Obese children are at a higher risk for heat disorders than normal-weight children.
- Be patient with regard to weight- and physical-activity-related expectations.
- Teach children to feel good about themselves, regardless of talent, body size, or shape.

- Be a role model: Eat a balanced diet and maintain a healthy body weight.

Parents
- Work with a health professional who has experience with weight control and young athletes to develop a medically sound and nutritionally balanced plan for your child.
- Encourage and support recommendations made by the health professional.
- Do not single out the obese child in the family by serving special foods or imposing restrictions. Include the whole family in making healthier, low-fat choices.
- Make mealtime pleasant. Encourage the child to eat slowly and to enjoy whatever he or she eats.
- Never give foods as a reward or withhold them as a punishment.
- Do not tell a child he or she is "on a diet" and that certain foods are "good" and others are "bad."
- Involve the child in shopping and food preparation.
- Never discuss the child's weight in front of others.
- Ask the advice of a health professional on the issue of other siblings or friends teasing the obese child.
- For the entire family, discourage eating meals and snacks while watching television.
- Examine your own dietary intake and attitudes toward food, and take an active role in establishing a healthy outlook toward exercise, eating, and body image with your child.

13

THE ACTIVE WOMAN: SPECIAL CONSIDERATIONS

WOMEN ARE VULNERABLE TO A VARIETY of social, economic, and emotional stigmas associated with their weight. It is difficult to feel good about oneself in a society that rewards thinness and scorns people who are overweight—particularly when the overweight person is a woman. Under the influence of this strong cultural bias for thinness, many women are unhappy with their body size and shape, believing that they are never thin enough. This fear of fatness drives large numbers of women to live their lives on a continuous quest to lose weight.

The constant struggle to control weight can cause many women, particularly active ones, to engage in a variety of disordered eating patterns. We'll discuss these, and their health risks, in the next chapter. At the very least, a woman's disrupted body image and disordered eating behavior perpetuate ongoing feelings of failure and poor self-esteem.

Many female athletes and active women believe that restricting their food intake will help them train better, and perform better, in addition to enhancing their overall appearance. Actually, restricting food intake to improve performance can cause depleted fuel stores, muscle wasting, weakness, fatigue, stress fractures, and impaired performance. Though some women manage to exercise well for a while without an obvious decline, injuries and lack of energy will eventually catch up with them.

Society as a whole needs to be educated about healthy weight and realistic body image. Young women, in particular, should be encouraged to develop a sense of self-esteem and self-worth that is not based solely on their body shape and size. This will help them to resist the pressure to conform to unrealistic and unattainable standards of appearance.

Women (and men) who have been repeatedly unsuccessful at weight-loss attempts may want to consider abandoning weight loss as a goal altogether. Instead of dieting, they can focus on normalizing their eating behaviors, eating more healthfully, becoming more physically active, and building positive self-esteem.

Active women, as active men, need to consume adequate carbohydrate and fluids. However, two minerals—calcium and iron—are of special concern to women. Nutritional deficiencies of either mineral can impair a woman's ability to exercise and possibly lead to health problems.

WOMEN'S NEED FOR CALCIUM

Calcium, the most abundant mineral in the body, is critical for the conduction of nerve impulses, heart function, muscle contraction, and the operation of certain enzymes. The bones and teeth contain 99% of the body's calcium; the remaining 1% circulates in the bloodstream. When the supply of calcium in the blood is too low, the body withdraws calcium from the bones.

An inadequate supply of calcium is one of the major contributing factors to osteoporosis, a disease that affects one in four women over the age of 65 and many women under 65 years.

Osteoporosis

Osteoporosis is an age-related disorder in which bone mass decreases and the susceptibility to fractures increases. Estrogen loss and inadequate calcium intake contribute to osteoporosis. Weight-bearing exercise and resistance training enhance skeletal calcium absorption and increase the strength of the bone, thus exerting a protective effect against osteoporosis.

Osteoporosis is a major public-health problem in the United States, affecting an estimated 24 million people and at least 25% of women after menopause. Every year, 1.3 million osteoporotic women over age 44 fracture one or more of their bones. Of those who sustain hip fractures, up to 20% die of complications, and many others lead altered lives due to chronic pain, disability, and depression. Economically, the direct and indirect annual costs of treating osteoporotic individuals range from $7 to $10 billion.

Because of their lower bone mass, women are more susceptible to osteoporosis. Also, after menopause women produce less estrogen, which further accelerates bone loss. Osteoporosis is called the "silent disease" because it usually is not detected until a fracture occurs, often in the hip, wrist, or spine. Dual X-ray absorptiometry is an accurate way to measure bone mineral mass with minimal radiation exposure.

Until peak bone mass is attained at approximately 30 to 35 years of age, bone formation exceeds the rate of bone resorption. The amount of bone mass a woman has by age 35 will strongly influence her susceptibility to fractures in later years. Therefore, calcium is as important to adults, especially adult women, as it is to children. The RDA for calcium is 800 mg per day for adult men and women, but the current RDA for women up to age 24 is 1,200 mg per day.

The National Institutes of Health (NIH) recommends that premenopausal adult women consume 1,000 mg per day. Women of any age who are on estrogen-replacement therapy should also consume 1,000 mg per day since they can still lose bone mass. Postmenopausal women who are not on estrogen should consume 1,500 mg per day.

The Health and Nutrition Examination Survery found that 50% of all females age 15 and over consume less than three-fourths of the RDA of 1,200 mg and that 75% of women over age 35 consume less than the RDA of 800 mg. The prevalence of calcium deficiency among women becomes even more serious in light of claims by the NIH and nutrition experts that the calcium needs of women actually are well above the recommended 800-mg level.

Obtaining Adequate Calcium

Dairy products represent the best sources of calcium. An 8-ounce glass of milk or ⅓ cup of nonfat powdered milk each contains about 300 milligrams of calcium. Skim or low-fat versions of milk, yogurt, cottage cheese, or cheese provide the same amount of calcium as the regular versions of these foods, but they contain less fat and calories.

Other good sources of calcium are sardines (because of the bones) and oysters. Broccoli and greens (kale, collard, turnip, and mustard) are good sources of calcium without any fat. Tofu that has been processed with calcium sulfate can also be a good source of calcium. Table 13-1 lists sources of calcium and the milligrams of calcium each provides.

Many factors determine how much calcium the body absorbs. For example, high intakes of protein, sodium, and caffeine interfere with calcium retention by increasing the amount of calcium excreted in the urine. Excessive alcohol intake has detrimental effects on bone mass. Inactivity, common among the elderly, also speeds calcium loss.

Should women take calcium supplements? Before opting for a supplement, consult a registered dietitian or physician for advice on how to obtain the appropriate amounts from food, and when appropriate, from supplements.

Too much calcium can be detrimental. In some people, excessive calcium intake increases the risk of urinary tract stones. Therefore, calcium intake should not exceed recommended levels.

TABLE 13-1
Sources of Calcium

	MG
MILK AND DAIRY PRODUCTS	
Milk, nonfat	*300*
Low-fat fruit-flavored yogurt	*345*
Low-fat plain yogurt	*415*
*Cottage cheese, 2%	*138*
*Cheddar cheese, 1 oz	*204*
*Mozzarella, part skim, 1 oz	*183*
*Parmesan, 1 oz	*390*
Ricotta, part skim, 1 oz	*77*
*Swiss, 1 oz	*272*
Tofu, 3½ oz	*127*
FISH	
*Salmon, canned, 3 oz	*167*
*Sardines, canned, 3 oz	*326*
WATER	
"Hard" water, 1 qt	*100*
"Soft" water, 1 qt	*30*
NUTS, LEGUMES	
Almonds, ½ cup	*173*
Lentils, cooked	*50*
Dried beans, cooked	*90*
VEGETABLES	
Certain leafy green vegetables,	*280*
including dandelion greens,	
mustard greens, turnip greens,	
collards and kale,	
but excluding spinach,	
beet greens, and chard	

All quantities are 1 cup unless indicated otherwise. Some good sources of calcium are also high in sodium, indicated with an asterisk (*). If you are not restricting sodium too much, you can still include these in your diet.

■ **Source:** *Maximize Your Body Potential*, by Joyce D. Nash, Ph.D., Bull Publishing Company, Palo Alto, CA. Used with permission.

Calcium carbonate (Tums or a generic equivalent) is an inexpensive and acceptable calcium source. Calcium carbonate is 40% calcium, so a 500-mg tablet actually provides 200 mg of elemental calcium. Such antacids that contain calcium are practically the same as dietary supplements. The primary difference between the two is in the marketing: When calcium carbonate is marketed as a calcium supplement, it costs more.

Bone meal and dolomite should not be used as calcium supplements because they may contain harmful amounts of lead, arsenic, mercury, and other potentially toxic minerals.

ATHLETIC AMENORRHEA

Some women who exercise strenuously stop menstruating, a condition called *athletic amenorrhea*. It is associated with low body weight/low body fat, nutritional inadequacy, physical stress and energy drain, and acute and chronic hormonal alterations. Although the specific cause of athletic amenorrhea is unknown and may vary among women, it appears to coincide with decreased estrogen production. When the athlete participates in a low-body-weight sport, the amenorrhea may be the result of disordered eating—the *athletic female triad*. Because estrogen deficiency is an important risk factor for the development of osteoporosis, amenorrhea may predispose female athletes to early-onset osteoporosis and fractures.

Spinal bone mass has been found to be lower in amenorrheic women runners compared to normal women runners. Especially disturbing is that further follow-up of these women indicated that bone mineral density remained well below the average for their age group four years after the resumption of normal menstruation.

It is not recommended that amenorrheic women athletes stop exercising. In fact, exercise may partially overcome the calcium withdrawal from the skeleton associated with estrogen deficiency. Women who have athletic amenorrhea should consult a physician to rule out any serious medical problems, and all amenorrheic women should consume 1,500 mg of calcium daily.

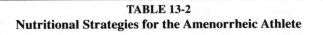

TABLE 13-2
Nutritional Strategies for the Amenorrheic Athlete

- *Reduce training*
- *Increase calories*
- *Increase calcium to 1,500 mg/day if not on estrogen-replacement therapy; otherwise, 1,200 mg/ day*
- *Try to gain weight*

After consultation with a physician, several strategies may be recommended to promote the resumption of menstruation. These include estrogen-replacement therapy, weight gain, diet modification, and reduced training. Table 13-2 summarizes nutritional strategies for amenorrheic athletes.

Regardless of menstrual function, most female athletes need to increase their calcium intake to meet the RDA for calcium.

WOMEN'S NEED FOR IRON

Iron-deficiency anemia is the nation's most common nutritional deficiency, affecting approximately 40% of women between the ages of 20 and 50. Iron is needed to form hemoglobin, an iron-containing protein that carries oxygen in the blood and releases it to the tissues. When the total hemoglobin concentration drops, the muscles do not receive as much oxygen. Table 13-3 shows the progression of iron deficiency to anemia.

Hemoglobin levels below 12 gm/dL for women and below 14 gm/dL for men are considered diagnostic for anemia. An anemic person has less endurance and cannot exercise as strenuously because the aerobic capacity is reduced due to the decreased oxygen-carrying capacity of the blood.

Women, compared to men, are much more likely to suffer from iron-deficiency anemia. Iron deficiency in women is usually

TABLE 13-3
Progression of Iron Deficiency to Anemia

PROGRESSION	METHOD OF DETECTION	HEMATOLOGIC PROFILE
Iron depletion	Serum ferritin	Depletion of iron stores in liver, bone marrow, and spleen
Iron-deficiency erythropoiesis	Serum iron, total iron-binding capacity, transferrin saturation	Depleted iron stores, decreased levels of plasma iron, increased hepatic formation of transferrin
		Increase of total iron-binding capacity to 400–500 mcg/dL
		Fall of percent transferrin saturation from mean of 30% to about 15–18%
Iron-deficiency anemia	HGB, RBC count hematocrit, mean cell hemoglobin concentration	Fall of hemoglobin concentration to below 12 gm/dL

■ **Source:** Adapted from *Physician Sportsmed.*, 1984.

the result of menstrual blood loss and inadequate dietary iron intake. There is also evidence that strenuous training accelerates the destruction of red blood cells, possibly due to mechanical trauma (such as hitting the ground while running) and gastrointestinal bleeding. Exercise increases the iron lost in sweat and appears to decrease iron absorption from the gut.

As we have seen from earlier material on vitamins and minerals, adequate iron intake is essential. The RDA for iron is 15 mg for women, but the average woman consumes only 10 mg per day. There are many ways to increase iron intake and correct this deficiency.

Obtaining Adequate Iron

Animal sources of iron should be emphasized, since the iron from them is better absorbed than the iron from vegetable sources. Combining animal and vegetable products (such as a meat-and-bean burrito) increases the iron absorbed from the vegetable product. Vitamin C also enhances iron absorption, so high vitamin C foods (e.g., orange juice) should be consumed with foods containing iron (e.g., iron-fortified cereals) for optimal absorption.

Cast-iron cookware also increases the iron content of foods. The more acidic and the longer the food is cooked in cast-iron cookware (e.g., spaghetti sauce), the higher the residual iron content of the food.

Red meat is an excellent iron source, containing about 1 milligram of iron per ounce. Iron-enriched or fortified cereal/grain products can contribute significantly to the iron content of the diet. Beans, peas, split peas, and some dark-green leafy vegetables are also good vegetable sources of iron. Table 13-4 lists sources of iron and the milligrams of iron each provides.

Because obtaining 15 mg of iron each day is a difficult task, and because many women are concerned about anemia, the supplement question again arises. Self-supplementation of iron is particularly dangerous. That "tired, listless feeling" can be caused by numerous conditions. Iron deficiency can be determined only by testing the blood for serum ferritin (storage iron) and checking the hemoglobin level.

Those women at risk for iron deficiency, particularly young menstruating female athletes, should have their hemoglobin levels checked periodically. A more sensitive, but expensive, test for iron deficiency also measures serum ferritin. Low ferritin levels appear in the first stage of iron deficiency, representing inadequate iron stores in the bone marrow. This test is valuable because it detects iron depletion early, before iron-deficiency anemia develops. A low ferritin level can mean that the person has an increased risk for developing iron-deficiency anemia. This allows iron stores to be increased through a greater intake of iron to head off the consequences of anemia.

TABLE 13-4
Sources of Iron

FOOD	MEASURING UNIT	IRON (MG)
*Liver-pork	3 oz	17.7
*Liver-lamb	3 oz	12.6
*Liver-chicken	3 oz	8.4
*Liver-beef	3 oz	6.6
*Oysters, fried	3 oz	5.9
Tostada, bean	1	3.2
Dried apricots	½ cup (12 halves)	3.0
Baked beans with pork and molasses	½ cup	3.0
Soybeans, cooked	½ cup	2.7
*Beef	3 oz	2.7
*Beef enchilada	1	2.6
Raisins	½ cup	2.5
Lima beans, canned or fresh cooked	½ cup	2.5
Refried beans	½ cup	2.3
Dried figs	½ cup (4 figs)	2.2
Spinach, cooked	½ cup	2.0
*Taco-beef	1	2.0
Mustard greens, cooked	½ cup	1.8
Corn tortilla, lime treated	8 inch diameter	1.6
Prune juice	½ cup	1.5
Peas, fresh cooked	½ cup	1.4
Enchilada, cheese and sour cream	1	1.4
Egg	1 large	1.2
*Turkey, roasted	3 oz	1.1
Sardines, canned in oil	1 oz (2 medium)	1.0

* Note: Foods of animal origin. Iron in foods of animal origin (except milk, which has little iron) is absorbed twice as efficiently as iron in foods of plant origin.
■ **Source:** *Food for Sport*, by Nathan J. Smith, M.D., and Bonnie Worthington-Roberts, Ph.D., 1989. Bull Publishing Company, Palo Alto, CA. Used with permission.

Iron supplementation will not improve the health or performance of a woman with normal iron stores. On the other hand, excessive intake can produce an iron overload (especially in a person who absorbs too much iron) and cause deficiencies of the trace minerals copper and zinc.

It is wise to consult a physician before taking an iron supplement. If iron supplements are used, they shouldn't exceed the RDA unless medically indicated and prescribed by a physician.

NUTRITION FOR EXERCISING PREGNANT WOMEN

Weight Gain

Adequate nutrient intake is essential during pregnancy to preserve the mother's body tissues as well as for the growth and development of the fetus. Appropriate weight gain during pregnancy is associated with increased infant birth weight. Also, prenatal malnutrition increases the incidence of neurological damage and mental retardation in the infant, since the fetal period is the initial phase of brain cell development.

An appropriate weight gain for exercising pregnant women is the same as that for sedentary pregnant women: from 24 to 28 pounds. The weight should be gained according to a definite pattern throughout the pregnancy. Two to four pounds should be gained in the first trimester. During the second and third trimesters, there should be a gain of approximately one pound per week.

Weight loss should never be attempted during pregnancy. Restricting weight gain can cause low-birth-weight infants, which is associated with an increased risk of infant death. When calories are restricted, the mother's protein intake, even if adequate, will be used for energy rather than for fetal growth. Also, ketosis, a condition that occurs when maternal fat stores are catabolized for energy, can cause serious abnormalities in the infant's central nervous system.

Energy Requirements

The caloric requirements of exercising pregnant women are unknown, although they may be estimated. The RDA for women of child-bearing age is 2,000, plus 300 calories for the daily cost of pregnancy, plus the additional calories needed to support exercise. Exercising pregnant women must obtain enough calories to provide energy for themselves, their fetus, and their activity. Not all pregnant athletes do this. Women who continue to exercise throughout pregnancy should be encouraged to consume adequate calories. As pregnancy progresses, it will take more calories to do the same weight-bearing activities, due to increased body weight.

Protein

Pregnant women should consume a total of 60 grams of protein per day. Exercise may also increase the protein requirement. However, the usual protein intake in this country exceeds recommended levels. Also, the increased food intake with pregnancy should provide adequate protein to meet the additional needs of exercising pregnant women.

Minerals

During pregnancy, the mother requires 15 mg of iron/day in addition to her nonpregnant RDA of 15 mg/day to increase her hemoglobin and to transfer necessary iron to the fetus. Iron from dietary iron sources or from the limited maternal iron stores is insufficient to supply the amounts needed for pregnancy. Pregnant women should receive 30 mg of elemental iron each day both to meet the need of the pregnancy and to protect their always-borderline iron reserves.

Iron needs may also be increased with endurance exercise. Iron stores—as measured by serum ferritin—are low in women runners, even with recommended iron intakes. This needs to be considered when determining if a pregnant woman may need more supplemental iron, above the 30 mg/day recommended. There is no evidence that iron supplementation during pregnancy causes an iron overload or is in any way harmful.

Pregnant women should consume 1,200 mg/day of calcium. This can be supplied by consuming a quart of milk or equivalent dairy products daily. This will also help to meet the added protein needs of pregnancy. If dairy products are not consumed, a calcium supplement should be taken.

Vitamins

Vitamin needs are higher during pregnancy. In general, B vitamin needs will be met by increased food intake. However, it is difficult to obtain enough folic acid from food during pregnancy since the requirement during pregnancy, 400 mcg, is twice the normal RDA for folic acid. A folic acid supplement of 400 mcg is recommended. This amount recently has been shown to reduce the risk of fetal neural tube defects, such as spina bifida (bulging of the spinal cord and/or meninges through a gap in the vertebral column) and anencephaly (absence of the brain). The fat-soluble vitamins and vitamin C can usually be obtained from dietary sources. In general, a prenatal vitamin and mineral supplement is recommended during pregnancy to ensure that all nutrients are adequately supplied to the fetus and to help prevent complications to the fetus.

Fluid Intake

Sedentary pregnant women should consume at least 8 cups (64 ounces) of fluids daily. Exercising pregnant women, especially those in hot environments, need to consume more. During exercise, women should drink at least 4 to 8 ounces of a rapidly absorbed beverage—water or sports drink—every 15 minutes. When women are not exercising, milk and juices are good fluids. Coffee and tea should be restricted by pregnant women due to their caffeine content. Consumption of alcohol during pregnancy can cause birth defects or other problems. Pregnant women should avoid alcohol completely.

14

EATING DISORDERS: THE SILENT DILEMMA

FOR ATHLETES, PARTICULARLY WOMEN, THINNESS is at a premium. Achieving the "ideal" image of the gaunt, emaciated body type is taking a costly toll. The tragic story of a world-class gymnast recently grabbed national attention. The headlines read: "She was tough, but the lure to be thinner was tougher. A U.S. gymnast dieted and starved herself until her body which had twirled and tumbled through a world championship meet—dwindled to 52 pounds. She was dead at 22 years" (*Philadelphia Inquirer*, July 26, 1994).

Losing weight in pursuit of the ideal weight or lean appearance becomes an all-consuming obsession for some athletes. As a result, eating behaviors evolve that jeopardize training, performance, and most important, health. Although recognition of these life-threatening disorders is growing, appropriate intervention and treatment for athletes lags far behind the problem.

PREVALENCE

The prevalence of eating disorders in athletes is estimated to vary from 1–39%. This reflects differences in the athletic population investigated, data-collection methods, and whether the diagnosis is based on self-reports or clinical interviews.

Though most studies have used surveys to establish prevalence, the validity of self-reports is questionable. Athletes may believe they can be identified from questionnaire responses. Even when anonymity is guaranteed, athletes can be reluctant to respond truthfully for fear of being discovered and losing their position on the team. This may explain why some studies show increased levels of eating problems and others do not.

Despite these limitations, it is assumed that eating disorders and their symptoms are more prevalent among female athletes than among female nonathletes or males. The incidence is higher among athletes competing in sports that emphasize leanness for enhanced performance (runners, wrestlers, lightweight crew) or for appearance (gymnasts, figure skaters, divers, ballet dancers).

DEFINITIONS AND DIAGNOSTIC CRITERIA

According to the revised fourth edition of the *Diagnostic and Statistical Manual of Mental Disorders* (DSM-IV-R, American Psychiatric Association, 1994), eating disorders are characterized as severe disturbances in eating behavior. The diagnostic criteria for these disorders are defined below.

- *Anorexia nervosa* is characterized by refusal to maintain body weight at or above a minimally normal weight for age and height; a distorted body image (the person "feels fat" even when emaciated); an intense fear of gaining weight or becoming fat while being underweight; and amenorrhea (the absence of at least three consecutive menstrual cycles).
- *Bulimia nervosa* is characterized by binge eating (rapid consumption of large amounts of food in a short period of time)

followed by inappropriate compensatory behavior to prevent weight gain such as self-induced vomiting; misuse of laxatives, diuretics, or enemas; fasting; or excessive exercise. The binge eating and inappropriate compensatory behaviors both occur at least twice a week for at least three months, and self-evaluation is unduly influenced by body shape and weight.

- *Eating disorder not otherwise specified (NOS)*. The disorders in this category do not meet the criteria for a specific eating disorder. Examples of NOS include individuals who binge-eat infrequently and individuals who have all the features of anorexia nervosa but have regular menses or a normal body weight.
- *Anorexia athletica*. An attempt has been made to identify the group of athletes who show significant symptoms of eating disorders but who do not meet the DSM IV-R criteria for anorexia nervosa, bulimia nervosa, or NOS. The classic features of anorexia athletica are an intense fear of weight gain or becoming fat even though the individual is lean, weight loss accomplished by a reduction in energy intake (often combined with exercise), and restrictive energy intake below that required to maintain high training volume. Binge eating is common, and such athletes frequently use pathogenic methods of weight control such as vomiting, laxatives, and diuretics. Some athletes with anorexia athletica also meet the criteria of NOS. Table 14-1 lists the diagnostic criteria for anorexia athletica.

RISK FACTORS FOR EATING DISORDERS IN ATHLETES

It is important to be aware of the expectations, performance demands, and factors that may place athletes at increased risk for eating disorders. This helps to facilitate early identification and treatment. The vulnerable athlete may be at high or low risk for an eating disorder depending on many sport-specific factors or demands.

TABLE 14-1
Diagnostic Criteria for Anorexia Athletica

ABSOLUTE CRITERIA	RELATIVE CRITERIA

Weight loss
  More than 5% of expected body
  weight
No medical illness or affective disorder
to explain weight loss
	Delayed puberty
	  No menstrual bleeding at age 16
	  (primary amenorrhea)

Excessive fear of obesity	*Menstrual dysfunction*
	  Primary amenorrhea, secondary
	  amenorrhea, oligomenorrhea

Food restriction *< 1,200 kcal/day*	*Gastrointestinal complaints*
	Distorted body image
	Purging *Self-induced vomiting, laxatives, diuretics* *Binge eating* *Compulsive exercise*

■ **Source:** Adapted from J. Sundgot-Borgen, Eating disorders in female athletes, *Sports Med. 17 (3): 176–188, 1994.*

Cultural Factors

Adolescents, especially women, are faced with enormous pressure to be thin and have an aesthetically pleasing appearance. Young women are continually bombarded with the message via fashion magazines and the media that having the "perfect body" symbolizes success, self-control, mastery, acceptance, and other values that are highly regarded by society.

For the adolescent female, changes in body composition such as increased body fat may be disconcerting even though this is a natural part of the maturation process. The inability to control weight and body shape may lead to a sense of frustration, guilt, and despair. Sports-related pressures and expectations go beyond the physical and emotional challenges already faced by athletes, particularly adolescent women. These stressors may initiate the development of a pattern of unhealthy eating that sets the stage for an eating disorder.

Psychological Factors

The behavior and attitudes of individuals with eating disorders and some athletes can overlap. Though high self-expectation, persistence, independence, perfectionism, competitiveness, and being goal-oriented may lead to excellence in the athletic arena, these qualities may also help to perpetuate an eating disorder. When an athlete with a vulnerable predisposition initiates a rigorous diet to manipulate body weight, it may become a self-perpetuating, self-reinforcing process.

Attraction to Sports and Exercise

Sport participation may attract individuals who already have characteristics of eating disorders, at least in personality and attitude if not in behavior or weight. For the eating-disordered athlete, abnormal eating and dieting behavior can be hidden or legitimized through sports. The athlete may try to "blend in" with others who are trying to meet the stereotyped standards of body shape in certain disciplines.

Competitive Status

It is not clear whether elite athletes are at greater risk than nonelite athletes. It can be argued that risk factors such as perfectionism and fear of failure may be more pronounced among elite athletes, increasing the risk for an eating problem. Or, as the athlete attempts to become elite, other pressures escalate and extreme measures may be taken to reach a higher goal.

Does exercise induce eating disorders? It has been theorized that exercise suppresses appetite, which serves to decrease the value of food as a reward. As a result, food consumption decreases and body weight is reduced. As weight decreases further, the drive for more exercise increases.

Although this theory has some support, not all individuals with anorexia nervosa exercise, and this theory does not explain bulimia nervosa.

Early Training

Having a certain body type may steer an individual toward a particular sport. For example, an adolescent who is tall and has a large frame would be more likely to opt for volleyball or basketball where height and size are viewed as an advantage, rather than opting for gymnastics where short stature and leanness are beneficial. Depending on the sport, the more the athlete's body deviates from the perceived ideal weight and body type, the higher the risk for an eating problem as the athlete struggles to meet the "ideal."

Athletes with eating disorders have been shown to begin sport-specific training significantly earlier than athletes who don't have eating disorders. Early training before maturity may prevent an athlete from choosing a sport more naturally suited to adult body type. However, in sports where thinness is emphasized such as gymnastics and figure skating, there is a strong trend toward an ever-younger group of athletes who may complete their amateur career prior to puberty or shortly thereafter.

Dieting and Weight Fluctuation

Periods of restrictive dieting and weight fluctuation have been suggested as important risk factors or triggers for the development of eating disorders in athletes. *Weight cycling* usually occurs in athletes who compete at a weight that is lower than their natural body weight. For example, a college wrestler weighs 155 pounds during the off-season but competes at 134 pounds in college.

Weight fluctuations occur during the season when the athlete struggles to achieve a low weight before competition, only to gain weight afterward when restraint weakens or other physiological processes promote restoration of a natural higher body weight. Other athletes cycle between seasons when weight is kept chronically below normal body weight for the competitive season and regained during the off-season.

Injury, Illness, or Loss of Coach

Some athletes have shown dramatic weight loss after losing or changing a coach, or following unexpected illness or injury. These circumstances may be viewed by athletes as a threat to continued success in their sport and may trigger an eating problem. Sexual abuse has also been reported as another possible explanation for the development of eating disorders among females. Unfortunately, there are documented cases of abusive relationships between male coaches and female athletes.

Athletes who have a fear of failure or performance anxiety may use an injury or decline in performance related to an eating disorder to justify disqualification or dismissal from the team.

Weight Expectations: Coaches, Trainers, Parents

It is not clear what impact weight-related expectations have on a young success-oriented athlete. Dieting has been shown to act as a trigger for extreme weight loss. However, if the athlete receives guidance on how to lose weight, the risk of developing an eating problem may be minimized.

In some sports, coaches may not convey a healthful attitude about body weight because of the demand for the athlete to meet a certain weight class (wrestlers) or achieve a certain appearance (gymnasts, figure skaters, ballet dancers, divers). Pressure to

TABLE 14-2
Complications of Anorexia Nervosa

• *Malnutrition*	• *Hypometabolism*
• *Loss of body fat*	• *Constipation*
• *Intolerance to cold*	• *Brain abnormalities*
• *Decreased muscle mass*	• *Amenorrhea*
• *Abdominal pain*	• *Sleep disorders*
• *Retarded gastric emptying*	• *Osteopenia*
• *Hypomotility, atrophy of GI tract*	• *Osteoporosis*
• *Excessively dry skin*	

reduce weight by coaches has been proposed as an explanation for the development of some eating disorders among athletes.

Coaches themselves do not traditionally induce eating disorders in athletes. However, inappropriate coaching or a lack of understanding about weight and body composition may trigger an excessive response in an individual who is susceptible to an eating disorder. Similar misunderstanding or weight-related demands may also come from family, friends, or teammates.

COMPLICATIONS OF EATING DISORDERS

Coaches, trainers, parents, health professionals, and athletes themselves must be aware of the potential medical complications of eating disorders. All too often, signs of eating disorders are ignored or minimized until serious medical complications occur. Tables 14-2 and 14-3 highlight key medical complications of anorexia nervosa and bulimia nervosa.

For the young athlete, the pressure to be thin may compromise normal growth. Athletes with eating disorders (except for some bulimics) consume suboptimal calories and nutrients to sustain physical activity and normal development.

Endocrine (hormonal) abnormalities have been well documented in anorexia nervosa, and more subtle endocrine abnormalities have been described in bulimia nervosa. Maintenance of a low body weight has been linked to delayed onset of menstruation and

---

TABLE 14-3
Complications of Bulimia Nervosa

VOMITING
- *Salivary-gland enlargement*
- *Lacerations of the oral cavity*
- *Esophageal inflammation*
- *Esophageal tears and ruptures*
- *Aspiration pneumonia*
- *Dental erosion*
- *Malnutrition*
- *Electrolyte disturbance:*
  mental confusion, hypokalemia
- *Cardiac arrest from: syrup of ipecac ingestion, hypokalemia*

DIURETICS
- *Dehydration*
- *Fatigue*
- *Poor skin turgor*
- *Electrolyte disturbance: hypokalemia, muscle cramps and weakness, headache, heart*
  palpitations, cardiac arrhythmia

LAXATIVES
- *Dependence on laxatives*
- *Diarrhea, constipation*
- *Bloating, gas, cramping*
- *Cathartic colon: incapable of peristalsis, thinning and atrophy*

---

amenorrhea. Amenorrhea is often accompanied by growth retardation and delayed onset of puberty. Many women with bulimia nervosa experience irregular menses, but frank amenorrhea is uncommon. Menstrual dysfunction also has been shown to be associated with scoliosis (abnormal lateral curvature of the spine) and stress fractures in young ballet dancers.

Unhealthy weight-loss practices through dehydration by water restriction, laxatives, and diuretics have potentially dangerous consequences. Fluid loss and accompanying electrolyte disturbances can increase the risk of an irregular heart rhythm, kidney damage, impaired temperature control, and loss of endurance and coordination. Gastrointestinal complications such as inflammation of the esophagus, esophageal tears, and inflammation of the pancreas can occur with bulimia nervosa. Fasting causes a decline in muscle and liver glycogen, which is detrimental to performance.

RECOGNITION OF EATING DISORDERS

The cornerstone of an eating problem is secrecy and denial, making identification and treatment a challenge. Weight-loss and dieting rituals in athletes do not always indicate an eating disorder. It is important to distinguish between behaviors associated with sports-induced requirements and the existence of an actual eating disorder. A clinical assessment by a health professional that includes detailed questions about exercise and nutrition, combined with perceptive interpretation of physical findings, is necessary to diagnose an eating disorder.

Unusual eating patterns or behaviors may come to the attention of staff and coaches through concerned team members who have noticed symptoms in a teammate. The coach may also observe decrements in performance and erroneously attribute them to a lack of effort or concentration. Whereas excessive weight loss is the most prominent clue to the recognition of anorexia nervosa, the athlete suffering from bulimia nervosa can appear healthy. Recognition of the problem may occur only with discovery of associated behaviors of bingeing and purging.

Key symptoms of eating disorders are presented in Table 14-4. These symptoms do not in themselves signify that an eating disorder exists, but several signs justify the need for further examination by a health professional. Coaches and trainers should use the following guidelines when faced with a suspected eating disorder in an athlete. (Adapted from Rosen and colleagues, *Phys. Sports. Med.*, 1986.)

1. Arrange a private meeting with the athlete. Under no circumstances should the athlete be spoken to about eating behaviors in front of a teammate.
2. Be direct and supportive in stating your concern. Tell the athlete specifically what behaviors/symptoms led you to think there is a problem.

TABLE 14-4
Physical and Behavioral Features of Eating Disorders

PHYSICAL FEATURES

- *Weight too low for athletic performance*
- *Precipitous weight loss*
- *Extreme fluctuations in weight*
- *Bloating or edema*
- *Swollen salivary glands, puffy cheeks or jaw just in front of ear*
- *Amenorrhea*
- *Proclivity to stress fractures*
- *Loss or thinning of the hair*
- *Sores or calluses on knuckles or back of hand from induced vomiting*
- *Muscle cramps*
- *Gastrointestinal complaints*
- *Headaches, dizziness, weakness due to electrolyte disturbances*
- *Numbness, tingling in limbs*

BEHAVIORAL FEATURES

- *Excessive dieting*
- *Excessive eating without weight gain*
- *Excessive exercise that is not part of the training program*
- *Guilt about eating*
- *Claiming to feel fat at normal weight*
- *Preoccupation with food, calories, and weight*
- *Denial of hunger*
- *Hoarding food*
- *Frequent weighing*
- *Evidence of binge eating—food wrappings, etc.*
- *Likely self-induced vomiting—bathroom visits just after heavy meals, etc.*
- *Use of drugs to control weight—laxatives, diet pills, diuretics, emetics*
- *Mood swings*
- *Avoiding food-related social activities*
- *Relentless, excessive exercise*
- *Wearing baggy, layered clothes*

■ **Source:** Adapted from D.M. Garner and L.W. Rosen, *J. Appl. Sports Sci. Res.* 5:100–107, 1991.

---

3. Make certain the athlete understands that the discussion is confidential.
4. State your concerns for that athlete as a person—not as the star player on the team. Health and well-being take precedence over her role as an athlete.

5. Address any concerns the athlete has about the eating disorder affecting sports participation. Reassure the athlete that training and competition will be limited only if there is evidence that performance is compromised to an extent that may lead to injury or that health is seriously threatened.
6. If the athlete admits that a problem exists, referral to a health professional (who is experienced with eating disorders in athletes) is essential for treatment.
7. If you strongly suspect that an eating problem exists and the athlete denies it, a mandatory meeting with a health professional for further evaluation is necessary. Explain to the athlete that pursuing help may be the single most important factor to achieve or preserve success in his or her sport.
8. Recognize that eating disorders are complex and treatment is a lengthy process. Show athletes that you understand their eating problems do not represent failure or a lack of effort.

There are several strategies that are important to *avoid* when approaching an athlete with an eating problem:

1. Never ignore the problem, hoping it will disappear with time. The problem will not correct itself and only becomes more serious and difficult to treat.
2. Never initiate a discussion with teammates about the problem. If you are approached by athletes, thank them for their concerns and reassure them that you will speak with the athlete privately.
3. The coach should never punish the athlete by dismissing her from the team or otherwise reprimanding her for an eating disorder. This will only make the athlete's eating problem worse.
4. Do not be reluctant to seek outside assistance from health professionals. Discussing the athlete's problem in confidence with a professional may be reassuring and will help you to determine treatment alternatives. Another possibility is to have a health professional give an informal talk about eating disorders to the team to discuss eating and weight-related

concerns. Educational materials can be handed out that highlight the symptoms and consequences of eating disorders and where the athlete can go to get help.

5. Never abandon the athlete after he or she agrees to seek treatment. Performance will most likely decrease during treatment, and expectations should be adjusted accordingly. This will minimize the anxiety the athlete already feels and will aid recovery.

PREVENTION OF EATING DISORDERS

Because the exact cause of eating disorders is unknown, it is difficult to determine preventive measures. It's important to heighten awareness to promote the early detection and treatment of eating disorders. Professionals who work with athletes *must* be educated about the risk factors for the development of eating disorders, their signs and symptoms, and their medical and psychological consequences.

Preventing the circumstances or triggers that may lead to an eating problem is critical. Many athletes who use rapid weight-reduction techniques do so under the assumption that weight loss will improve performance. However, the metabolic consequences of vomiting and laxative abuse have a negative effect on health and performance and can be fatal. Although there have been some notable exceptions in which athletes have performed successfully despite eating problems, they are exceptions. Athletes need to know that an eating disorder is a threat to health as well as performance.

Coaches and parents need to realize that their opinions and remarks about body weight can strongly influence an athlete's eating behaviors. Commenting on an athlete's body size or need for weight loss (without offering guidance on how to lose weight healthfully) may trigger the development of an eating problem in certain athletes who are at risk for eating disorders.

Realistic weight goals should be identified and agreed on by the athlete, health professional, and coach. Changes in body composition should also be monitored in relation to performance. Private weigh-ins are essential to reduce the anxiety and stress associated with traditional team weigh-ins. In an effort to achieve or maintain a reasonable competitive weight, nutritional counseling is necessary by a qualified sports nutritionist. The sports nutritionist can individualize guidelines for weight control and the athlete's sports-specific nutritional demands.

Finally, the sports community must consider the demand placed on athletes to achieve unrealistic weights and body shapes. When body composition standards for a sport seriously compromise the health of many athletes, it is a matter of grave concern for everyone involved. Where does the responsibility lie? With the athlete? With coaches? Sports judges? Parents? The media? All may play a significant role in placing a premium on thinness. How much longer can the well-being and performance potential of our athletes be threatened?

15

NUTRITION FOR THE CHILD ATHLETE

Participation in athletics often begins at an early age and has become an important part of growing up for many children. In addition to the health benefits associated with physical activity, exercise provides children with opportunities for personal enjoyment, social interaction, and skill development. Athletic participation can be used to introduce children and their families to sound nutritional practices that may provide an important lifelong health benefit. Parents and coaches need to consider the special needs of young athletes for training and performance. Table 15-1 provides the Young Athlete's Bill of Rights.

PHYSICAL GROWTH

All children should have their height and weight plotted by a health professional on the National Center for Health Statistics growth charts. These charts are routinely used by pediatricians

161

TABLE 15-1
Young Athlete's Bill of Rights

---

1. *The right to have the opportunity to participate in sports regardless of ability level.*
2. *The right to participate at a level commensurate with the child's developmental level.*
3. *The right to have qualified adult leadership.*
4. *The right to participate in a safe and healthy environment.*
5. *The right of each child to share leadership and decision making.*
6. *The right to play as a child and not as an adult.*
7. *The right to proper preparation for participation in sports.*
8. *The right to equal opportunity to strive for success.*
9. *The right to be treated with dignity by all involved.*
10. *The right to have fun through sports.*

■ **Source:** "So What's Good About Sports?" *Am J Dis Child* 1988; 142:143. © 1988 AMA. Reprinted with permission from the American Medical Association.

---

to evaluate growth of children and adolescents. Increases in height and weight during the early school-age years are small compared with the rapid growth observed during infancy and adolescence. Young children typically grow 2 to 3 inches and gain 3 to 6 pounds each year. At puberty, however, children undergo hormonal changes that mark the beginning of adolescence. These hormonal changes cause them to grow rapidly. It is especially important to make certain that children entering puberty are meeting their nutritional needs.

Tanner Stages of Development

The rate and age of sexual maturation is highly variable and differs within and between the sexes. To help monitor maturing children, the Tanner stages of sexual development (sexual maturity ratings) can be used (Table 15-2). This numerical system has been established for describing children in terms of how their bodies are changing and developing sexually.

Although formal Tanner staging is determined by a physician, other characteristics can be used to estimate the level of

TABLE 15-2
Tanner Stages of Development

STAGE		BOYS	GIRLS
1		Prepubescent	Prepubescent
2		First appearance of pubic hair	First appearance of pubic hair
	Peak Growth Spurt in Girls	Growth of genitalia	Development of genitalia
		Increased activity of sweat glands	Increased activity of sweat glands
3		Pubic hair extends to scrotum	Pubic hair thicker, coarser, curly
		Growth and pigmentation of genitalia	Breasts enlarge and pigmentation continues
	Peak Growth Spurt in Boys	Changes in voice Beginning of acne	Genitalia well developed Beginning of acne
4		Pubic hair thickens, facial hair begins	Pubic hair abundant, armpit hair begins
		Growth and pigmentation of genitalia	Breasts enlarge and mature
		Voice deepens	Genitalia assume adult structure
		Acne may be severe	Acne may be severe Menarche begins
5		Increased distribution of hair	Increased pubic hair distribution
		Genitalia fully mature	Breasts fully mature
		Acne may persist and increase	Increased severity of acne (if present)

sexual maturity. For girls, the rapid period of growth is completed when menstruation begins at Tanner stage 4. Boys grow fastest between stages 3 and 4. Following the growth spurt in stage 4, the boy has enough circulating hormones in the blood to facilitate muscle mass and show signs of facial hair. Upon examination, if a boy has only "peach fuzz" for facial hair and/or has not started shaving, he probably has not completed his growth spurt.

EATING BEHAVIORS AND PATTERNS

When a child reaches elementary school, he develops eating patterns that are more independent of the influence and scrutiny of his parents. New activities and friends begin to influence choices as the child is exposed to a variety of new foods and different social situations. School-age children tend to be repetitious in their food choices, and the food groups they include in their diets remain relatively constant from month to month.

Many school-age children skip breakfast. Usually, the main reason is lack of time. Children who eat breakfast may have a better attitude, school record, and problem-solving ability compared to children who do not eat breakfast. In addition, breakfast helps to replenish liver glycogen stores depleted during an overnight fast. This ensures that the child has adequate energy stores for afternoon training. Children should be encouraged to find foods they like for breakfast. These do not need to be traditional foods. Food composition, not social tradition, is the best strategy.

Some athletes such as figure skaters practice early in the morning before they go to school. Under these circumstances, the child should be encouraged to have a small snack before activity such as fruit juice and toast, followed by additional carbohydrate-rich foods and fluids afterward.

The child's lunch may be provided by the school or brought from home. The federal government requires its school lunch program to provide approximately one-third of the recommended daily allowances for children. Many changes have been implemented in the school lunch program in recent years. For example, popular items such as pizza, tacos, macaroni and cheese, and hamburgers are often included on the menu, fresh fruits are provided as an alternative to desserts like cake and cookies, and skim milk is offered in addition to whole milk.

School lunch is often more nutritious than a lunch brought from home. This is because box lunches typically contain less variety and include only favorite foods. In addition, they are limited to foods that travel well and do not require heating or refrigeration. Even if a nutritious lunch is packed at home, the parent does not necessarily know what portion is eaten, traded, or thrown away.

Food choices are typically influenced by the child's friends. To gain a better understanding of what the child eats, parents should ask children if they eat lunch with their friends and why they prefer certain foods.

Snacks may contribute significantly to the child's nutrient intake and eating style. The quality of snacks eaten may determine whether nutrient requirements are being met. Therefore, the frequency of snacking and type of snacks are important considerations. For example, does the child snack during the morning and/or before going to bed? What are the child's favorite snacks? Are they prepared at home or purchased from a vending machine?

For most athletes, practice is held after school. After a training session, many children come home from school exhausted and hungry. Bakery products, soft drinks, candy, and chips often top their list of favorites, and they are the most frequently chosen snack foods. It is important that nutritious foods, especially those quick and easy to prepare, are available at typical snack times. In addition, the child should be encouraged to rehydrate by consuming water and fruit juices.

DIETARY RECOMMENDATIONS FOR YOUNG ATHLETES

For the school-age child athlete, increased caloric needs for training are best met by planning daily intake around the Food Guide

Pyramid. This encourages consumption of a variety of foods that include all the necessary nutrients. The child should consume 2 to 3 servings of milk, 2 to 3 servings of meat/protein, 4 servings of vegetables, 3 servings of fruits, and 9 servings of bread/grains a day. This represents an intake of about 2,200 calories. The exercising child may need an additional 500 to 1,500 calories depending on the frequency, intensity, and duration of activity. Though foods containing fats or sugars are not eliminated, they should not replace essential items of the diet. These accessory foods should be consumed in moderation and in addition to, but not in place of, other foods.

The child should be encouraged to distribute food intake over regular periods of time throughout the day. This will ensure the presence of readily available sources of energy to support training activity. To be effective in getting the child to actually eat the recommended foods, it is important to suggest changes that are compatible with the eating habits of the child.

How Parents Can Help Their Children Eat Better

Parents can explain basic facts about the different food groups and how the foods relate to exercise. Attempts to teach children nutrition concepts and information should take into account their developmental level. For example, parents should explain that carbohydrate foods like bread and pasta provide energy for the muscles to work well and that dairy foods like milk help build strong bones. The objective here is to increase the child's awareness of good nutrition habits, not to enforce stringent guidelines at this age.

The school-age child relies for the most part on the foods that are brought into the house. In addition to the parent purchasing more healthful foods, favorite foods can be made more nutritionally dense or acceptable substitutions can be made with similar foods. There are many different food choices available that will supply adequate amounts of vitamins and minerals for even the choosiest of eaters.

Small changes that are acceptable to the child can be encouraged to increase nutrient density. For example, fortified cereals can be served rather than sugary ones, and peanut butter cookies can be offered instead of chocolate cream cookies. Parents can pack snacks and fluids for before and after practice so that the child does not have to rely on vending machines.

Variety and balance in the family menu will underscore the importance of eating different foods to provide the range of nutrients necessary for growth and development. Ideally, this is achieved by regularly scheduled meals at home plus nutritious snacks. However, this may not be possible. An important issue facing parents with children in sports is how to provide nutritious meals when there are hectic practice schedules. Workouts may interfere with home meals, resulting in a greater reliance on convenient fast foods or the child eating alone after the family has finished. Children need to be taught how to make nutritious food choices at fast-food restaurants since most popular choices are high in fat and salt and low in vitamins A, C, and fiber.

SPECIAL FLUID NEEDS OF CHILDREN

Children do not tolerate temperature extremes as well as adults. They produce less sweat yet generate more heat during exercise and are less able to transfer this heat from muscles to the skin. Relative surface area is greater for a child compared to an adult, which results in greater heat gain in extreme heat and greater heat loss in cold weather. Children also have a lower cardiac output.

Acclimatization to exercising in the heat is more gradual in children compared to adolescents or adults. A child may require 5 to 6 sessions to achieve the same degree of acclimatization acquired by an adult in 2 to 3 sessions in the same environment. From a practical standpoint, the intensity and duration of exercise should be restrained during the first 4 to 5 days a child begins an exercise program, particularly in the heat. Over a period of 1½ weeks, activity can be slowly increased.

All of the preceding factors increase the risk of dehydration in children. Therefore, fluids play a critical role in maintaining health and performance of the child athlete. Heatstroke ranks second among reported causes of death in high school athletes. By educating young athletes about how it occurs, heatstroke can be prevented. Because a substantial level of dehydration can be reached before an athlete ever feels "thirsty," special emphasis should be placed on ensuring adequate fluid intake in children and adolescents before, during, and after physical activity. Guidelines for fluid replacement are shown in Figure 15-1.

Fluid intake can be facilitated by providing athletes with a personalized bottle and encouraging them to drink 4 oz every 20 minutes of activity. Supervision of fluid intake is essential, particularly for children, because they do not instinctively drink enough fluid to replace water losses. During prolonged exercise, children and adolescents may not recognize the symptoms of heat strain and may push themselves to the point of heat-related illness. If the child tires easily and repeatedly in practice, appears irritable, and performance suddenly declines, dehydration and/or inadequate caloric intake may be the cause.

Plain water is the most economical source of fluid to hydrate the body. However, children may be more likely to drink sufficient amounts if they are given flavored fluids. A sports drink or diluted fruit juice (1 cup juice and 1 cup water) would be appropriate.

PREVENTING HEAT DISORDERS IN YOUNG ATHLETES

In addition to making sure that the young athlete drinks enough fluids, adults can take a number of precautions to significantly reduce the risk of heat injury in children:

- Adjust the timing of practice depending on weather conditions. Schedule workouts for the coolest time of the day (before 10 a.m., after 6 p.m.) especially in warm, humid

FIGURE 15-1
Fluid Guidelines for Young Athletes

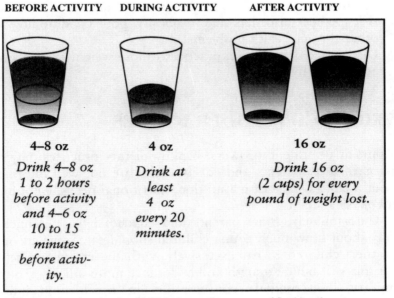

BEFORE ACTIVITY   DURING ACTIVITY   AFTER ACTIVITY

4–8 oz	4 oz	16 oz
Drink 4–8 oz 1 to 2 hours before activity and 4–6 oz 10 to 15 minutes before activity.	Drink at least 4 oz every 20 minutes.	Drink 16 oz (2 cups) for every pound of weight lost.

Kids ages 10 and under should drink the smaller amount of fluid listed.

■ **Source:** Adapted from F. Meyer and O. Bar-Or, *Sports Med.* 18 (1): 4–9, 1994.

weather conditions. Extreme heat and humidity are valid reasons to cancel practice or competition.

- Allow athletes to adjust to intensity of exercise sessions and warmer conditions gradually.
- When possible, avoid excessive clothing, taping, or padding on hot/humid days. For example, on such days, schedule football workouts with padding and other gear for early morning instead of afternoon.
- Schedule frequent water and rest breaks in the shade. Insist that all athletes drink a certain amount of fluid before returning to practice.
- Never withhold water as a disciplinary measure. Water should be available at all times of training and competition.

- Because volume of sweat loss varies, weigh athletes before and after exercise to estimate total water loss during practice.
- Be aware of children and adolescents who may be at increased risk for heat disorders due to obesity, poor conditioning, or other chronic health problems.
- Discourage dehydration practices to lose weight and encourage proper hydration.

WEIGHT-CONTROL PRACTICES

In pursuit of athletic prowess, healthy dietary practices may be disregarded by parents and coaches who are not well informed about a child's stage of maturation, nutritional needs, emotions, and physical ability.

Unfortunately, some parents and coaches have misconceptions about how much young children should eat. Some encourage their children to eat excessively, with the erroneous belief that this will build strength and endurance more quickly. To the contrary, indiscriminate consumption, in which food intake exceeds the child's caloric requirement, may be the start of a life-long struggle with being overweight.

At the other extreme are parents who adopt a restrictive diet that may endanger the health of the child. Given the current focus on lowering cholesterol and fat, many parents may encourage their children to do the same in an attempt to minimize the future risk of heart disease. However, the American College of Pediatrics Committee on Nutrition does not recommend low-fat diets for young children. Rather, it recommends that children receive 30% of total calories from fat. Restriction of intake to lower levels may hinder adequate growth and development.

Diets restricted in fat and cholesterol often reduce the intake of cheese, meat, and milk, which are major sources of protein, iron, calcium, and other minerals necessary for growth. Parents can encourage long-term healthful habits without compromising growth needs by offering foods with moderate amounts of unsaturated fat versus foods high in saturated fat.

For some sports, weight-related demands on athletic children by a parent or coach can be sudden and extreme, such as running laps during hot weather to eliminate excess body fat. Food intake may also be chronically restricted in an effort to enhance performance. Fatigue, heat exhaustion, and illness can result. Nutritional needs for growth and development must be placed before athletic considerations.

SUPPLEMENTS

Young athletes can meet their vitamin and mineral needs on diets that include the foods and servings recommended in the Food Guide Pyramid. Vitamin, mineral, or protein supplements are not recommended for healthy child athletes. Unfortunately, many well-meaning (but misinformed) parents and coaches advise children to take supplements in an effort to promote early athletic development and improve performance and as "nutrition insurance." However, eventual maturity and athletic ability do not depend on how early children begin adolescence. Growth will not be facilitated by promoting the use of dietary supplements.

Children need to understand that taking large doses of vitamins and minerals can be dangerous. Providing children with supplements can give them a false sense of security and may encourage faulty eating habits. They may assume that their morning dose of supplements provides them with all the nutrients they need so that they can eat candy and soda instead of cereal and milk.

Another disadvantage of supplement use is that child athletes may erroneously associate improvements in performance with whatever supplements they may happen to be taking. They may be less likely to attribute progress to training, hard work, and a balanced diet. This type of false reinforcement may also encourage children to try other types of supplements and substances (including steroids), which can lead to a snowball effect with undesired consequences. Aside from being dangerous, large doses of nutrients do not make up for a lack of training or talent nor do they give athletes a competitive advantage.

To move away from this reliance on "supplement insurance," young athletes need to feel confident about eating "ordinary foods." Parents, coaches, and health professionals must emphasize how regular foods promote muscle growth and optimal performance. From a practical standpoint, this is an important reason to encourage young athletes to keep records of what they eat, how they train, and how their performance improves. These records can be used to illustrate the importance of good dietary and training habits as the cause of improvement, rather than leaving the child to erroneously associate athletic accomplishments with a pill.

If children understand why extra vitamins and minerals are unnecessary (and potentially dangerous), they will learn to refrain from using them at an early age and continue to do so during adolescence when peer pressure is amplified. For the young athlete, the key to health and performance cannot be found in any one food or supplement. Instead, a proper combination of foods provides the many different nutrients the body requires. Variety and moderation is the best strategy to achieve balance.

16

NUTRITION FOR
THE OLDER
ATHLETE

OLDER ATHLETES, AS ALL ATHLETES, must consume adequate dietary carbohydrate and fluid to ensure optimal athletic performance. Regardless of age, the athlete should have a diet that helps to reduce the risk of chronic diseases such as coronary heart disease, stroke, and cancer.

HEART-HEALTHY TRAINING DIET

Masters athletes can obtain a healthy, high-performance diet by following the U.S. Dietary Guidelines. As shown in Figure 16-1, carbohydrates (predominantly complex) should provide at least 60% of total calories, fat no more than 30% of calories, and protein at least 12% of calories. Dietary fat should provide less than 10% of total calories as saturated fat, up to 10% unsaturated fat, with monounsaturated fat making up the difference. Cholesterol intake should be limited to 300 mg or less daily.

FIGURE 16-1
The Current U.S. Diet and the Recommended Diet

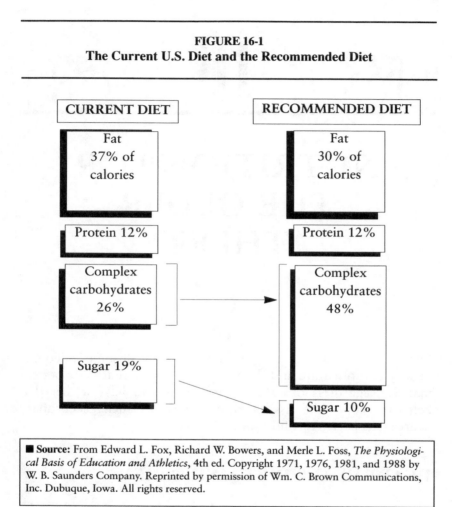

| CURRENT DIET | RECOMMENDED DIET |

Fat 37% of calories → Fat 30% of calories

Protein 12% → Protein 12%

Complex carbohydrates 26% → Complex carbohydrates 48%

Sugar 19% → Sugar 10%

Most older athletes will need to decrease their fat intake (an average of 37% of calories) and increase their carbohydrate intake (from an average of 45% of calories) to 6–8 gm of carbohydrate per kg/day. The U.S. Department of Agriculture's Food Guide Pyramid and National Cholesterol Education Program's Step 1 diet can provide practical dietary guidelines for older athletes.

Consuming more servings of complex carbohydrates and fruit will increase consumption of dietary fiber as well as carbohydrate. At the very least, a high-fiber intake helps to relieve constipation, a common problem of sedentary older people.

A low-fat, high-fiber diet may help to prevent diverticular disease, colon cancer, and coronary heart disease. Eating fruits and vegetables rich in vitamin C and beta-carotene may also reduce the risk of certain cancers.

VITAMINS AND MINERALS

Although vitamin requirements do not appear to change with age, sedentary older individuals may not consume adequate amounts due to low caloric intakes. While little is known about the effects of physical activity on vitamin requirements in older athletes, a varied diet should cover any increased needs associated with exercise. Fortunately, older athletes tend to eat more than their sedentary peers and so tend to get more vitamins and minerals in relation to their needs.

Ensuring adequate dietary consumption of vitamins D and B_{12} is important among older adults. Frequently observed low levels of vitamin D among the elderly may be attributed to several factors, including suboptimal sunlight exposure, age-associated changes in metabolism of vitamin D, and/or medications that may influence metabolism. If the athlete is involved in an outdoor sport, exposure to sunlight should be adequate.

Despite sufficient amounts of vitamin B_{12} in the diet, some individuals are unable to absorb B_{12} because they lack the gastric enzyme called intrinsic factor. Gastric, intestinal, and pancreatic disease can lead to intrinsic-factor deficiency. An adequate consumption of low-fat animal products should ensure adequate vitamin B_{12} blood levels, as long as absorption is not hindered.

Older athletes who consume nutrient-poor diets or take in fewer than 1,500 calories a day may benefit from a vitamin/mineral supplement containing no more than 100% of the recommended dietary allowances (RDAs). When therapeutic doses of vitamins are indicated because of increased requirements due to drug interactions or metabolic dysfunction, the individual must be carefully monitored. Older individuals may be more susceptible to vitamin/mineral overload and so should be discouraged from taking self-prescribed doses of any vitamin or mineral exceeding the RDA.

Age is associated with a reduced requirement for some minerals, so supplements are typically not warranted. For example, the poor iron status of many women usually vanishes following menopause. As with vitamins, if the dietary intake is adequate, proper iron, zinc, and copper status will be maintained despite strenuous training.

Calcium is an important mineral in the diets of older athletes because of its relationship to bone density. The skeletal calcium loss incurred by older people, especially women, can lead to stress fractures and osteoporosis. Estrogen replacement and adequate calcium intake can reduce the bone mineral loss that occurs as women age. Exercise is also beneficial by retarding calcium loss from the skeleton and promoting a greater calcium intake due to a greater caloric intake. Although the RDA is 800 mg, the National Institutes of Health suggests that post-menopausal women obtain 1,000 mg of calcium per day when on estrogen-replacement therapy and 1,500 mg per day when untreated.

BODY COMPOSITION AND WEIGHT CONTROL

The energy requirements of the sedentary individual will decrease over time due to the loss of fat-free mass (primarily muscle), which declines by 15% between the third and eighth decades of life. However, prudent resistance training can help preserve muscle mass and reduce the age-related decline in metabolic rate.

Also, because the energy required for exercise does not change with age, physical activity can help to slow or abolish the age-related decline in caloric needs. This enables the older athlete to more easily maintain a desirable body composition, while enjoying a higher caloric and nutrient intake.

As with younger athletes, the energy needs of the older athlete should be determined based on age, type of activity, and time spent exercising.

HYDRATION AND HEAT TOLERANCE

As people get older, their ability to remain properly hydrated decreases due to a decreased sensation of thirst and changes in kidney function. As with younger athletes, the first side effect of dehydration is impaired performance. However, this may be followed by the more serious consequences of heat exhaustion, heatstroke, or even death.

Compared to younger adult athletes, older athletes respond to excessive heat with higher body core temperatures and heart rates, lower sweating rates, and an overall greater loss of body water. However, these differences don't necessarily translate into poorer heat tolerance during exercise.

The primary measures of heat tolerance (changes in core temperature and heat storage) show minimal age-related declines when older men and women maintain a high degree of aerobic fitness. The ability to exercise in a hot environment is less a function of age than of aerobic fitness and health status.

Maintaining proper hydration during exercise is important for both performance and health. Thus, older athletes should be especially careful to drink fluids according to a time schedule (4 to 8 ounces every 15 minutes) rather than according to thirst, since their perception of thirst is diminished.

17

SUPPLEMENTS AND NUTRITION QUACKERY

"NEW PERFORMANCE BREAKTHROUGH! Makes more energy available to your muscles. Increases your speed and strength without additional training. Our unique supplement is an energy-releasing substance extracted from natural foods by a secret process. Send $49.95 for your starter capsules now!"

But first, keep your hand on your wallet.

If you read a typical fitness magazine, you know that there is no shortage of nutrition supplements which supposedly increase speed, enhance endurance, relieve muscle soreness, improve muscle mass, or reduce body fat. Some advertisements even claim their wonder product does all of the above.

Athletes seek that "secret ingredient" which will enhance their workout and give them the edge over their competitors. As a result, they are susceptible to nutrition quackery. Many athletes resort to nutritional supplements as performance-enhancing aids. However, if you're looking too hard for the magic bullet, you may find it in places it doesn't exist.

You can avoid being a victim of a nutrition rip-off by learning to recognize the techniques nutrition quacks use to manipulate consumers. When you observe any of the following—stop, take a deep breath, and keep your money in your pocket.

WARNING SIGNS

The claims sound too good to be true, but they are what people want to hear. Nutrition quackery is successful because quacks play on emotions and misinformation. Most athletes want to believe there are "magical" alternatives to the hard training and sound diet that promote improved performance. However, they are rarely told of possible side effects or other harm that might result from the promoted product or dietary regimen.

Quacks encourage distrust of reputable health professionals such as medical doctors, registered dietitians, and other nutrition scientists. They ridicule the nutrient content of our food supply and claim that the foods we need to meet nutritional requirements can't be purchased in grocery stores. They refer to their unproven treatments as "alternatives" to reputable medical care. Though choices do exist among current legitimate treatments, the alternatives promoted by quacks can be ineffective and/or unsafe.

Quacks often use case histories, testimonials, and subjective evidence to justify their exaggerated claims. Quacks try to appear trustworthy by having well-known athletes promote their product. Testimonial evidence is by definition biased and uncertain. Scientists report their studies in reputable journals, where their work is reviewed and evaluated by other scientists prior to publication. Controlled experiments that can be confirmed by repeating the study are the best way to document the accuracy of the information.

Evaluating Claims

You need to be discriminating about the nutrition information you read and hear. Most victims of nutrition fraud aren't gullible, only unsuspecting. Magazines, books, and the media overflow with medical advice—some reliable, some inaccurate.

Here are some guidelines you can use to evaluate nutrition claims:

- *What are the qualifications of the person recommending the product or diet?* A reputable person usually has a background or current affiliation with an accredited university or medical school offering programs in the fields of nutrition or medicine. Beware the title "nutritionist." It can be used by anyone, regardless of training. Even "Ph.D." is no guarantee. Sad to say, a quack can purchase the credential from a diploma mill (an unaccredited institution) to appear legitimate.

- *What evidence does the person supply for any claims that are made?* The claims should be supported with references to the scientific journals that published the original research. Is the information factual and specific or vague and highly emotional? Are the recommendations based on published scientific evidence or on personal testimonials?

- *If the information is written, why was it published? Is someone trying to sell you something?* Does the material encourage gradual changes in your lifestyle, or does it promise to dramatically enhance performance or guarantee fast results? Does the author recommend eating a variety of foods, or are certain foods eliminated? Are expensive supplements recommended as the only way to ensure nutritional adequacy?

- *Do the suggestions appear to agree with most recommendations of medical and sports science professionals?* Professional journals review articles in a wide range of lay publications and judge their credibility. If you don't have access to these—and most athletes don't—you can seek the advice of a registered dietitian or other qualified nutrition professional at a local university, health department, or hospital. If you're considering big changes in eating habits that have kept you healthy until now, this extra digging is worthwhile.

OTHER STRATEGIES QUACKS USE

Quacks are clever at imitating health professionals and scientists. When quacks assess a person's nutritional status, they use various "tests" to diagnose nutritional deficiencies and food allergies. They use these tests to appear scientific, convince people to buy nutrition supplements, or even to profit directly from the cost of the test. The tests used by quacks include cytotoxic testing, applied kinesiology, live cell analysis, iridology, and hair analysis.

Using fake tests, these fake nutritionists always find something wrong. Their typical "diagnoses" include: food allergies, hypoglycemia, malabsorption, glandular disturbances, adrenal insufficiency, trace vitamin and mineral deficiencies, and the build-up of various toxins in the body. These are all problems that sound ominous and are difficult to prove or disprove with a fake test.

Quacks may claim they are doing a nutrition assessment—but what makes up a valid nutrition assessment? A nutrition assessment may be part of a general health examination and requires the combined expertise of a medical doctor and a registered dietitian. It generally includes a medical history, dietary history, and clinical evaluations. If neither a registered dietitian nor a physician is involved, you should be suspicious.

Quackery is very subtle. Fitness-oriented people want to believe in something that is magical which can improve performance more than hard training or a prudent diet. In many events the difference between winning and losing is split seconds, so it is not surprising that athletes are susceptible to claims for magical foods or nutrients.

The placebo effect by itself is powerful enough to produce beneficial results. When athletes are convinced that certain products improve performance, their belief may enable them to perform better, even though there is nothing useful in the product as such. Just because a friend may ride the placebo effect to a better performance, it doesn't mean you will.

Most of the time, quacks do injury only to our wallets, promising benefits they can't deliver. However, they can cause real harm when necessary medical treatment is delayed at a time when it could be most effective in treating an illness or injury.

ERGOGENIC AIDS

Ergogenic aids represent the trendiest area in sports nutrition. They supposedly enhance performance above levels anticipated under normal conditions. Ergogenic means "work producing." Many athletes believe that certain ergogenic aids will give them a competitive edge. In fact, many offer no benefits, and some are harmful.

Ads for such products often display muscular individuals and/or endorsements from body-building or weight-lifting champions. Locker conversations about "bulking up" also perpetuate nutrition myths and misinformation.

There are several reasons that athletes believe various products have helped them. The use of the product often coincides with natural improvement due to training. Also, increased self-confidence or a placebo effect inspires greater performance. This "psychological benefit" should be weighed against the dangers of misinformation, wasted money, misplaced faith, and adverse side effects that can result from use of some of these products.

There is no scientific research to back up the claims made for most of these products. Unfortunately, athletes, as well as the general public, often believe that advertisements and testimonials are proof of effectiveness.

Currently popular ergogenic aids (other than protein, amino acids, and vitamins) that have not been scientifically proven to be effective include the following:

- *Boron* (a trace element that influences calcium and magnesium metabolism). Claim: Increases serum testosterone levels, thereby increasing muscle growth and strength. Fact: Boron has no effect on testosterone levels, lean body mass, or strength in strength-trained athletes.
- *Carnitine* (a compound synthesized in the body from the amino acids lysine and methionine). Claim: Increases fat

metabolism and decreases body fat. Fact: Carnitine facilitates the transfer of fatty acids into the mitochondria (the energy powerhouses of the cell) where they are burned for fuel in the aerobic energy system. There is no evidence that carnitine supplementation increases the use of fatty acids during exercise or decreases body fat. There is no dietary requirement for carnitine.

- *Choline* (precursor of the neurotransmitter acetylcholine and a component of lecithin, a substance involved in fat transport). Claim: Increases strength (by increasing acetylcholine) and decreases body fat (by increasing lecithin). Fact: There is no dietary requirement for this substance, and a deficiency has never been demonstrated in humans. The body can manufacture choline from methionine, an essential amino acid. There is no evidence that increasing choline intake will increase strength or decrease body fat.

- *Chromium* (an active component of the glucose tolerance factor, which facilitates the action of insulin). Claim: Increases muscle mass, decreases body fat, and promotes weight loss. Fact: Two unpublished studies conducted by one researcher suggest that chromium picolinate supplementation during weight training increases muscle mass and decreases body fat. This same researcher holds the patent on chromium picolinate, and unfortunately, patenting laws do not require that claims for health products be valid. Also, the studies had several major methodological weaknesses that make their results questionable. Independent research does not support the claims that chromium supplements increase muscle mass, decrease body fat, promote weight loss, or have any value as an alternative to anabolic steroids.

- *Coenzyme Q10* (a catalyst in the aerobic energy system). Claim: Optimizes ATP production to increase energy and stamina. Fact: There is no dietary requirement for this substance, and a deficiency has never been demonstrated in humans. Supplementation with coenzyme Q10 does not improve endurance performance or aerobic capacity.

- *Gamma-Oryzanol* (a plant sterol derived from rice bran oil). Claim: Increases serum testosterone and growth hormone, and increases muscle growth without the side effects of anabolic steroids. Fact: Like other plant sterols, gamma-oryzanol isn't ergogenic because it can't be converted to testosterone by the human body.
- *Ginseng* (extract of ginseng root). Claim: Increases energy, increases resistance to stress and disease, and cures almost everything. Fact: No other drug has all the healthful properties attributed to ginseng. The existence of a genuine cure-all is unlikely. Until proper research is conducted, the claims for ginseng should be considered unproved. Because ginseng is expensive, the commercial preparations may have little or no ginseng. Though the best-documented side effects of ginseng are insomnia and, to a lesser extent, diarrhea and skin eruptions, the prolonged use of ginseng appears to be relatively safe.
- *Glandulars* (extracts from animal glands such as adrenals, pituitary, testes). Claim: Enhance function of the same gland in the human body; for example, testes extract enhances testosterone production. Fact: These glandular extracts contain no hormones and so can't exert an anabolic effect on the body. If they could, they would be dangerous for self-medication.
- *Inosine* (a nucleoside involved in the formation of purines). Claim: Increases ATP production, increases strength, and enhances recovery. Fact: There are no performance benefits from consuming inosine. Inosine is broken down during digestion and does not reach the body's cells intact.
- *Lecithin* (phosphatidylcholine). Claim: Prevents fat gain. Fact: Lecithin is a phospholipid. Phospholipids are powerful emulsifying agents and so are essential for the digestion and absorption of fat. Although lecithin has a role in the digestion of dietary fat, it has no effect on body fat. The body produces an ample amount of lecithin, and supplementation is unnecessary.
- *Lipotropic factors* (include carnitine, coenzyme Q10, arginine, and ornithine). Claim: Increase fat loss with exercise. Fact: See comments under appropriate sections.

- *Medium chain triglycerides, or MCTs* (fats that are water-soluble and readily absorbed). Claim: Promote muscularity and body fat loss, increase thermic effect. Fact: MCTs are ineffective as a fuel source during aerobic exercise. There is no proof that MCTs increase muscularity or enhance body fat loss in strength-trained athletes. Consuming large amounts can cause gastrointestinal upset and diarrhea.
- *Metabolic bars* (such as PR Bar). Claim: Eating metabolic bars and following a strict dietary regimen (40% carbohydrate, 30% protein, and 30% fat) increase fat metabolism and promote body fat loss. Fact: There is no evidence that metabolic bars improve fat metabolism or decrease body fat above and beyond the effects of exercise training. Athletes who follow the dietary regimen may have impaired performance due to low muscle glycogen stores.
- *Omega-3 fatty acids* (polyunsaturated fatty acids found mostly in fish oils). Claim: Stimulate release of growth hormone. Fact: Omega-3 fatty acids may be converted to prostaglandins (hormonelike-substances) in the body. A specific prostaglandin called PGE 1 does stimulate growth hormone release. There is no proof that omega-3 fatty acids improve aerobic endurance or have an ergogenic effect in strength-trained athletes.
- *Pangamic acid* (also referred to as vitamin B_{15}. Its composition varies, depending on supplier). Claim: Increases delivery of oxygen. Fact: Pangamic acid is not even a single substance—different sellers put different synthetic ingredients in a bottle. Pangamic acid products provide no health or performance benefit and have contained compounds that could cause cancer or other adverse effects.
- *Smilax* (a genus of desert plants containing several species of sarsaparilla). Claim: Naturally increases serum testosterone levels, thereby increasing muscle growth and strength—a legal alternative to anabolic steroids. Fact: Though Smilax does contain substances called saponins that can serve as precursors for the synthetic production of certain steroids, this conversion takes place only in the laboratory, not in the human body. There is no evidence that

Smilax is anabolic or functions as a legal replacement for anabolic steroids. The saponins in Smilax have a diuretic and laxative effect.

- *Succinate* (a metabolite in the aerobic energy system). Claim: Enhances metabolism, reduces lactic acid, and maintains ATP production. Fact: Succinate is an intermediary in the aerobic pathway. Supplemental succinate will not "speed up" the process of aerobic metabolism or ATP production as this is controlled by enzymes within the pathway.
- *Superoxide dismutase* (enzyme). Claim: Protects the body against oxidative cell damage incurred from aerobic metabolism. Fact: Superoxide dismutase is an antioxidant enzyme found in most body cells. It works with other antioxidants such as vitamins C and E to protect the cells from oxidation. No benefit for humans has ever been demonstrated. This is because oral superoxide dismutase is digested and does not reach the bloodstream intact.
- *Vitamin B_{12}* (essential for DNA synthesis). Claim: Enhances DNA synthesis and increases muscle growth. Fact: Since vitamin B_{12} is essential in the synthesis of DNA, the claim is that enhancing DNA synthesis stimulates muscle growth. Dibencobal (a form of B_{12}) is advertised to increase muscle growth. There is no evidence that Dibencobal or vitamin B_{12} promotes muscle growth or enhances strength.
- *Yohimbine* (an alkaloid extracted from yohimbine bark that increases serum levels of norepinephrine). Claim: Increases serum testosterone levels, increases muscle growth and strength, and decreases body fat. Fact: There is no proof that yohimbine is anabolic. Documented health hazards include low blood pressure, weakness, and nervous stimulation, followed by paralysis, fatigue, stomach disorders, kidney failure, seizures, and death.

The following are ergogenic aids that have scientific support for their effectiveness.

- *Caffeine* (an alkaloid stimulant found in coffee, tea, and some medications that increases serum levels of epinephrine).

Claim: Improves performance. Fact: Consuming 5–9 mg of caffeine per kg before exercise may improve performance during endurance exercise and short-term intense exercise lasting about 5 minutes. The use of caffeine is considered a form of doping by the International Olympic Committee (IOC). The IOC has set an upper limit of 12 micrograms per milliliter of caffeine in the urine. Theoretically, the IOC threshold would be reached by consuming 8 cups of coffee (at 100 mg/cup), 4 tablets of Vivarin, or 8 tablets of No-Doz.

Whether it is ethical to use this drug to enhance performance is an issue requiring individual evaluation and judgment. Potential side effects of caffeine ingestion include nausea, muscle tremors, palpitations, and headache. In hot weather, the diuretic effect of caffeine could contribute to inadequate rehydration following exercise.

- *Creatine* (combines with phosphate to form creatine phosphate, or CP, a high-energy compound stored in muscle). Claim: Increases CP content in muscles, increases energy, and stimulates muscle growth. Fact: Preliminary research suggests consuming 20 to 25 grams of creatine increases power in short-term, high-intensity exercise up to 30 seconds. It also appears to increase body weight, due to gain of either muscle protein or water. Additional research is needed to confirm these benefits. If creatine is proved effective, the use of creatine supplements could be considered doping because this high amount can't be obtained through diet. As such, creatine supplements would violate the ethics of sport performance.
- *Sodium bicarbonate* (buffers lactic acid in the blood). Claim: Augments the body's buffer reserve, counteracts the build-up of lactic acid in the blood, and improves anaerobic performance. Fact: Several studies have supported improved anaerobic performance (400- and 800-meter runs) with bicarbonate administration. Taking 0.3 gm/kg of sodium bicarbonate with water over a 2- to 3-hour period may improve 800-meter run time by several seconds. However, as many as half of those using sodium bicarbonate experience urgent diar-

rhea one hour after the soda loading is completed. The effects of repeated ingestion are unknown, and caution is advised. Use of sodium bicarbonate may also be construed as doping, thereby breaching the ethics of sports performance.

- *Phosphates* (part of ATP and CP). Claim: Improved endurance. Fact: Phosphate loading may increase a compound called 2,3-DPG (2,3 diphosphoglycerate) in the red blood cells that facilitates the release of oxygen to the muscles. The increase in 2,3-DPG may increase aerobic capacity and decrease the rise of lactic acid during submaximal exercise. The dose is 1 gram of sodium phosphate, taken 4 times a day for 3 days. Use of phosphates may also be considered a form of doping, thereby violating the ethics of sports performance.

THE BOTTOM LINE

New ergogenic aids for athletes are constantly emerging. Often, these products are marketed without any supportive scientific research to indicate the potential benefits or possible harmful side effects. Prosecutions or other legal actions take years, and the promoter can reap huge profits during the delay.

Under U.S. consumer protection laws, a substance is considered a drug if a *medical claim* is made for it, even though it is a food or dietary supplement. However, just about anything can be sold as long as it is called a dietary supplement. Since the Food and Drug Administration treats dietary supplements as foods, these products are not evaluated for safety and effectiveness.

To help combat nutrition fraud, the Food and Drug Administration has mandated that, by July 1995, all nutrients in dietary supplements must be listed on the label. Although claims on the label cannot be false or misleading, supplement manufacturers often use advertising techniques such as testimonials and pamphlets that are protected by the First Amendment to the Constitution (freedom of speech).

The supplement manufacturers currently have the advantage—their products don't have to be safe or effective. People tend to believe that the products on the market have been researched, tested, and inspected. Americans, including athletes, are being bilked out of millions of dollars that would be better spent on food and training.

Athletes should avoid buying products with bogus claims like "fat burner," "fat metabolizer," "energy enhancer," "performance booster," "strength booster," "ergogenic aid," "anabolic optimizer," and "genetic optimizer."

Your best protection against nutrition fraud is to be an informed consumer. If you have questions about a particular supplement, contact a registered dietitian specializing in sports nutrition or the National Council Against Health Fraud, P.O. Box 1276, Loma Linda, CA 92354.

18

EATING ON
THE ROAD

OBTAINING A NUTRITIOUS HIGH-CARBOHYDRATE MEAL while traveling from one competition to another is a challenge. Meal stops are often made at fast-food restaurants because they're convenient and relatively inexpensive. However, a typical fast-food meal is often high in fat (and sodium) and low in fiber, calcium, and vitamins A and C.

This chapter provides recommendations for team travel, fast-food strategies, ideas for snacks at convenience and grocery stores, tips to decipher menus, recommendations for different cuisines, tips for packing a cooler, and other road-travel suggestions.

TEAM TRAVEL

It helps to determine where the team will eat before mealtime. This way, an establishment can be located that will provide a high-carbohydrate meal (such as spaghetti or pizza) within the

191

budget. Restaurant managers are generally accommodating, especially if notified in advance and if this becomes a regular request.

When the team is staying in a hotel that offers food service, the catering manager can be contacted to ask for high-carbohydrate meals that fit within the budget. Examples of high-carbohydrate breakfasts include pancakes or hot cereal with muffins, fruit juice, and low-fat milk. Lunch could consist of a turkey or chicken sandwich on whole-wheat bread, low-fat yogurt or ice milk, and fresh fruit. Dinner could be a pasta main course with bread, salad, fruit, and low-fat milk.

FAST-FOOD STRATEGIES

Breakfast is a good fast-food team meal choice due to the varied selection of high-carbohydrate foods: cereal (hot and cold), bagels, muffins, pancakes, toast, fruit, and fruit juices. (See Table 18-1 for low-fat fast-food choices.)

For example, at McDonald's, two whole English muffins with jam, 1 scrambled egg, 6 oz of orange juice, and one 8-oz carton of 2% milk provide 56% carbohydrate and 25% fat for a total of 747 calories. Hot cakes with butter and ½ packet of syrup, 6 oz of orange juice, and one 8-oz carton of 2% milk provide 66% carbohydrate and 25% fat for a total of 650 calories.

Many fast-food chains also offer high-carbohydrate lunch and dinner choices. At McDonald's or Carl's Jr, a barbecued chicken sandwich, a side salad (easy on the dressing), 6 oz of orange juice, and one 8-oz carton of 2% milk provide a meal that's about 50% carbohydrate and 25% fat for a total of 677 calories.

Compare this to a McDonald's Big Mac, which supplies 500 calories—47% from fat and only 34% from carbohydrate. A small order of fries adds 220 calories, of which 49% are fat. Combine the Big Mac and fries and you have 720 calories, 48% derived from fat.

At Wendy's, 8 oz of chili, a plain baked potato, a side salad (with vegetables and 1/4 cup cottage cheese), and a small shake

TABLE 18-1
Making Lower-Fat, Nutritious Fast-Food Choices

LOWER-FAT CHOICES	MODERATE-FAT CHOICES	HIGH-FAT CHOICES
Dairy Foods		
Low-fat milk	2% milk	Whole milk
Frozen yogurt	Soft-serve ice cream	Hard ice cream
Low-fat milk shakes	Milk shakes	
Starches		
Bagels, English muffins	Small order French fries	Biscuit, croissant
Pancakes, waffles	Cornbread	Hash browns
Cereals		Large order French fries
Bread sticks		Curly, cheese, or other fries
Baked potatoes		Pastry, pie, or brownie
Salad Bar		
Salad	Chicken, tuna salad,	Olives, croutons
Carrot, celery sticks	Cole slaw	Bacon bits
Pasta	Macaroni / potato salad	More than 2 tbsp. of dressing
Fresh fruit		Cream-based soups
Soups, not cream-based		
Low-fat dressings		
Meats / Main Dishes		
Chicken filet	Cheeseburgers	Fried chicken
Chicken fajita	Steak sandwiches	Fried chicken sandwich
Grilled chicken sandwich		Fried fish/fried fish sandwich
Chili with beans		Fish or chicken nuggets
Plain hamburgers		"Super," "deluxe," or
Vegetable pizza		"supreme" sandwich or
Chicken / turkey / ham / roast		burger
beef sandwich or sub		Sausage, pepperoni, or extra
Bean burrito		cheese pizza
		Bacon burger
		Breakfast biscuits (egg with
		sausage or steak)
		Sausage, bacon
Sauces		
Catsup		Mayonnaise
Mustard		Mayo-type sauces
Barbecue sauce		Alfredo sauce
		Hollandaise sauce
		Added butter or margarine

offer about 57% carbohydrate and 25% fat for a total of 1,016 calories. Baked potatoes can be substituted for french fries, and nonfat or low-fat milk can be substituted for a shake.

Mexican and pizza establishments are probably the best fast-food outlets for high-carbohydrate, low-fat meals. For example, at Taco Bell, two tostadas (plain shell, not fried), one bean burrito, two plain tortillas, and one 8-oz carton of 2% milk provide a meal that's about 56% carbohydrate and 27% fat for a total of 1,040 calories. Recently, low-fat versions of the original meals have been added to the menu.

At Pizza Hut, one-half of a medium thin-crust cheese pizza, two bread sticks, and an 8-oz glass of 2% milk supply about 56% carbohydrate and 25% fat for a total of 1,126 calories. Remember to choose vegetable pizza toppings to increase carbohydrate and reduce fat. Appendix A lists other fast-food breakfast, lunch, and dinner suggestions.

CONVENIENCE AND GROCERY STORE IDEAS

For athletes on a tight budget or seeking a variety of choices, a nearby grocery store can offer a variety of high-carbohydrate, low-fat foods—even a soup and salad bar. Many athletes stop at convenience stores for snacks while traveling. Distance cyclists often stop at these establishments to refuel—but if they're not careful, they may load up on more fat than carbohydrate. With this in mind, we'll take a stroll through a grocery store to evaluate some typical snacks.

A 2-oz bag of potato chips offers 306 calories, but 58% come from fat and only 38% from carbohydrate. By comparison, a 2-oz bag of corn chips has about the same amount of calories, but 43% come from carbohydrate and 51% from fat—less fat than potato chips but still higher than recommended.

Nuts and seeds, although full of nutrients, are even higher in fat and calories. Peanut butter supplies 95 calories per tablespoon—with 78% of calories from fat. Two ounces of roasted peanuts provide 344 calories. A whopping 73% of these are fat calories, whereas only 15% are carbohydrate. Likewise, 2 oz of almonds translates into 352 calories, of which 83% are fat and 13% are carbohydrate. Be wary of snacking on sunflower seeds: Two ounces provide 314 calories, 76% from fat and 14% from carbohydrate. For a crunchy high-carbohydrate snack try baked crackers, baked tortilla chips, rice cakes, low-fat granola bars, air-popped popcorn, or pretzels.

Cookies provide lots of calories, primarily from fat and sugar. For example, two large Pepperidge Farm chocolate chip cookies provide about 320 calories, of which 55% are carbohydrate but 41% are fat. Two large Pepperidge Farm oatmeal cookies provide 305 calories, of which 58% are carbohydrate and 38% are fat.

Fig bars would be a lower-fat selection. Two provide only 106 calories, 80% from carbohydrate and just 17% from fat. Because their calorie content is lower than that of most cookies, they're a good sweet snack choice for calorie-conscious athletes. Fat-free cookies, such as Snack-Wells, provide carbohydrate calories, but not fat calories.

Candy bars are a favorite snack choice. A Snickers provides 270 calories, 43% from fat and 49% from carbohydrate. Most candy bars contain about an equal proportion of fat and carbohydrate. Milky Way is an exception. Of its 260 calories, 66% come from carbohydrate and 31% from fat. Hard candies and licorice provide mainly carbohydrate calories and little or no fat. Table 18-2 lists some low-fat, high-carbohydrate candies.

Most pastry items contain more fat than carbohydrate due to added fat in frying or in fillings. For instance, a Hostess cake donut provides 115 calories, of which 44% is carbohydrate and 55% is fat. A regular raspberry danish twist provides 220 calories, 49% from fat and 49% from carbohydrate, compared to a fat-free raspberry danish twist that has 140 calories, none from fat and 94% from carbohydrate.

The bread aisle provides foods that are low-fat and packed with complex carbohydrates and B vitamins. Try bagels, whole-grain rolls and breads, raisin bread, english muffins, and pita bread.

TABLE 18-2
Low-Fat, High-Carbohydrate Candy

FOOD ITEM	SERVING SIZE	KCAL	CARBOHYDRATE	FAT
Bit-O-Honey	1.7 oz	200	78%	18%
Butterscotch discs (Brach's)	3 pieces (0.6 oz)	70	97%	0%
Candy corn (Brach's)	21 pieces (1.4 oz)	150	99%	0%
Caramels	2 pieces	60	80%	20%
Jelly beans (Brach's)	12 pieces (1.4 oz)	140	100%	0%
Gummy bears (Brach's)	5 pieces (1.4 oz)	130	99%	0%
Fruit Juicers (Life Savers)	2	80	100%	0%
Peanut brittle (Kraft)	1 oz	130	62%	34%
Peanut chews (Goldenbera's)	4 pieces (1.7 oz)	215	60%	29%
Skittles	1.5 oz	170	89%	11%
Starburst	8 pieces (1.4 oz)	160	83%	17%
Twizzlers	4 pieces (1.4 oz)	130	93%	7%
York Peppermint Pattie	1 (1.5 oz)	180	76%	20%

Though regular ice cream is high in fat, some related products are low in fat and calories. For example, whereas a Dove Bar provides 350 calories and 51% fat, an ice-cream sandwich supplies 167 calories, 62% provided by carbohydrate and only a third from fat. A popsicle or juice bar has no fat—all of its calories come from carbohydrate in the form of sugar.

Probably the best selection in the dairy aisle is yogurt. A cup of fruit-flavored low-fat yogurt is 225 calories, of which 75% come from carbohydrate and only 10% from fat. Low-fat or fat-free pudding and yogurt are also available and provide fewer than 225 calories, with carbohydrate and protein. Unlike ice cream, fruit bars, and popsicles, yogurt is nutrient dense with calcium, protein, and B vitamins. Low-fat cheeses and low-fat milk are other healthy dairy snacks.

It's easy to find high-carbohydrate items in the cold-drink section. Twelve ounces of soda supply 140 to 180 calories, all of which are carbohydrate in the form of sugar. A more nutritious carbohydrate alternative that's also 100% carbohydrate is fruit juice, which supplies, on average, 180 calories per 12 ounces. Other good choices are sports drinks containing 6–8% carbohydrate (about 60 to 80 calories per 8 ounces). If the goal is rapid replacement of fluid losses, they're a better choice than juices and sodas (see Chapter 9).

Fresh fruit is another healthy choice. Fruit is nearly 100% carbohydrate and supplies vitamins, minerals, and fiber. A banana provides about 120 calories, and an apple and an orange each supply about 60.

DECIPHERING RESTAURANT MENUS

When you are dining at restaurants, the menu offers many clues to the fat content of foods. Words such as fried, crispy, breaded, scampi style, creamed, buttery, au gratin, and gravy all suggest that another food item should be chosen. Better choices are items carrying such descriptions as steamed, broiled, boiled, char-broiled, poached, marinara, tomato sauce, and "in its own juice."

TIPS FOR DIFFERENT CUISINES

Mexican

At Mexican restaurants, chicken and bean burritos (not deep fried), soft tacos, and tostadas are good choices. When available, pot beans or black beans can be substituted for refried beans. (Some restaurants offer refried beans that are fat-free or made with vegetable oil instead of lard—ask your server.) Heated corn tortillas can be substituted for chips, and salsa can be substituted for sour cream (or ask for low-fat) and guacamole.

Here are some lower-fat Mexican choices:

Salsa
Gazpacho soup
Black, red beans
Spanish rice
Fajitas
Soft chicken, seafood tacos (flour, corn)
Refried beans (without lard)

Note that guacamole, sour cream, and cheese add fat. Low-fat or nonfat sour cream is a healthier choice.

Italian

At Italian restaurants, pasta is a good choice, but marinara sauce is recommended over alfredo and pesto sauces, which are high in fat. Thick-crust plain cheese or vegetable pizza is another good choice, as are salads with dressing on the side. Bread is great, but go easy on the butter or margarine. Low-fat italian ices are better choices than rich desserts.

Here are some lower-fat Italian choices:

Pasta with marinara, marsala, tomato sauce

Pasta with red clam sauce
Chicken marsala
Spinach tortellini
Minestrone soup
Bread sticks

Note that antipasto, fried calamari, breaded meats and eggplant, pesto, and fettucini alfredo are traditionally high-fat dishes.

Chinese

When dining at Chinese establishments, choose stir-fried and steamed dishes (such as rice) with plenty of vegetables. Avoid deep-fried items (egg rolls and wontons) and high-fat foods such as spare ribs and sweet and sour pork. Though low-fat selections are available, note the high sodium content in Chinese foods. To reduce excess sodium, ask that your food be prepared without monosodium glutamate (MSG, a flavor enhancer) and go easy on the soy sauce. One tablespoon of soy sauce contains 11 calories but 1,029 milligrams of sodium!

Here are some lower-fat Chinese choices:

Steamed rice
Chicken chow mein
Chicken/beef chop suey
Stir-fry with shrimp, vegetables, chicken
Hunan tofu
Hot and sour soup
Wonton soup
Fortune cookies

Note that stir-fries and sweet-and-sour dishes are often made with deep-fat–fried meats and shrimp. Fried chow mein noodles, fried rice, egg rolls, and lobster sauce (made with egg yolks) are "hidden" sources of fat. Chinese food is typically high in sodium.

Indian

Eastern foods, such as those from India, feature beans, fruit chutneys, rice, grains, vegetables, and bread, all of which are high in carbohydrate and low in fat. The food is often steamed, thus adding little fat. Watch dishes made with coconut milk and cream.

EATING WHILE TRAVELING

When embarking on long car, bus, train, or plane rides, many athletes load up on candy bars, chips, and soft drinks. Switching to pretzels, bagels, fruit, popcorn, granola bars, crackers, water, and sports drinks will provide less fat and more carbohydrate. Adding an ounce or two of low-fat protein foods, such as lean meat or mozzarella cheese, can make snacks more satisfying without increasing fat intake.

In fact, the coach or athlete can pack a cooler for bus or road trips. This will help to ensure that athletes have the proper fuel for competition. Foods that can be included in the cooler include bagels, flavored rice cakes, pretzels, fresh and dried fruits, carrots and celery sticks, graham crackers, animal crackers, fig bars, low-fat or nonfat yogurt, part-skim string cheese, turkey sandwiches, sports bars, liquid meals, fruit juices, and sports drinks.

Air travel presents some unique challenges. The pressurization of the cabin increases fluid losses, so dehydration can be a problem when the flight lasts several hours or longer. In fact, dehydration is thought to contribute to jet lag. Consuming beverages containing alcohol and caffeine increases the risk of dehydration because of the diuretic nature of these beverages. The athlete should emphasize nondiuretic fluids such as water and fruit juices to replace fluid losses.

Airlines don't always provide low-fat meals. However, low-fat or vegetarian meals are available when requested in advance. Athletes can also bring high-carbohydrate, low-fat snacks with them on the plane. If they don't receive a meal on the plane, they can purchase healthy snacks at airport concession stands, such as soft pretzels, popcorn (without butter), bagels, fruit/vegetable plates, juice, and frozen yogurt.

COACHING TIPS

Coaches and trainers are important role models for their athletes. Why stress the importance of good nutrition when the coach and trainer are on the sidelines drinking soda and eating french fries? To change the eating habits of athletes, those working with them should encourage them to make wise food choices, give them the opportunities to practice making good choices, and set a good example.

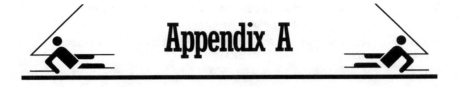

Appendix A

FAST-FOOD CHOICES FOR BREAKFAST, LUNCH, AND DINNER

THE FOLLOWING TWO TABLES, A-1 AND A-2, list lower-fat, high-carbohydrate breakfast, lunch, and dinner choices at selected fast-food restaurants.

TABLE A-1
High-Carbohydrate Breakfast Food Choices at Selected
Fast-Food Restaurants

FOOD ITEM	SERVING SIZE	KCAL	CARBO-HYDRATE	PROTEIN	FAT	EXCHANGES
CARL'S JR.						
English muffin with margarine	2 oz	190	63%	13%	24%	2 starch, 1 fat
Bran/blueberry muffin	4.8–4.2 oz	310–340	67–72%	13–14%	20–24%	3½ starch, 1 fat
Orange juice	9 oz	90	93%	7%	0%	1½ fruit
McDONALD'S						
Egg McMuffin	4.8 oz	280	40%	25%	35%	2 starch, 2 medium fat meat
Cheerios	¾ cup	80	70%	15%	15%	1 starch
Wheaties	¾ cup	90	84%	9%	7%	1 starch
Fat-free apple bran muffin	2.6 oz	180	89%	11%	0%	2½ starch
Hot cakes Syrup	1 order 1 ½ fl oz	250 120	80%	13%	7%	3 starch, ½ fat 2 fruit
Apple, grape-fruit, orange juice	6 oz	80	95%	5%	0%	1 fruit
ARBY'S						
Cinnamon nut danish	3.5 oz	360	67%	6%	27%	4 starch, 2 fat
Blueberry muffin	2.7 oz	240	67%	7%	26%	2½ starch, 1 fat

TABLE A-2
Lower-Fat, or High-Carbohydrate Lunch and Dinner Food Choices at Selected Fast-Food Restaurants

FOOD ITEM	SERVING SIZE	KCAL	CARBO-HYDRATE	PROTEIN	FAT	EXCHANGES
ARBY'S						
French dip sandwich	5.4 oz	368	38%	25%	37%	2 starch, 2 medium fat meat, 1 fat
Grilled chicken bar-becue sand-wich	7.1 oz	386	49%	21%	30%	3 starch, 3 medium fat meat
Hot ham and cheese sand-wich	6 oz	355	39%	26%	35%	2 starch, 3 medium fat meat
Light roast chicken deluxe sand-wich	6.8 oz	276	48%	46%	6%	2 starch, 2½ lean meat
Light roast turkey deluxe sandwich	6.8 oz	260	51%	42%	7%	2 starch, 2 lean meat
Roast chicken salad	14 oz	204	47%	22%	31%	1 starch, 2 vegetable, 1 medium fat meat
Light Italian dressing	2 oz	23	52%	0%	38%	½ fat
Baked potato	8.5 oz	240	83%	10%	7%	3 starch
Garden salad	11.6 oz	117	38%	24%	38%	2 vegetable, 1 fat
Lumberjack mixed veg-etable soup	8 oz	89	58%	12%	30%	1 starch
Old-fash-ioned chicken	8 oz	99	61%	21%	18%	1 starch

TABLE A-2
**Lower-Fat, High-Carbohydrate Lunch and Dinner Food Choices at
Selected Fast-Food Restaurants (continued)**

FOOD ITEM	SERVING SIZE	KCAL	CARBO-HYDRATE	PROTEIN	FAT	EXCHANGES
BURGER KING						
Hamburger	3.6 oz	260	43%	22%	35%	2 starch, 2 medium fat meat
BK Broiler Chicken sandwich	5.4 oz	280	41%	27%	32%	2 starch, 2 medium fat meat
Chicken salad without dressing	9 oz	142	23%	52%	25%	1 vegetable, 2 lean meat
Light Italian dressing	2 oz	30	80%	0%	20%	½ fat
Lemon pie	3.2 oz	290	68%	7%	25%	3 starch, 1 fat
CARL'S JR						
Hamburger	4.3 oz	320	41%	18%	39%	2 starch, 2 medium fat meat
Charbroiler BBQ chicken sandwich	11 oz	310	44%	39%	17%	2 starch, 3 lean meat
Teriyaki chicken sandwich	8.3 oz	330	51%	33%	16%	2 ½ starch, 2 ½ lean meat
Santa Fe chicken sandwich	7.8 oz	540	56%	22%	22%	5 starch, 2 ½ lean meat

TABLE A-2
Lower-Fat, High-Carbohydrate Lunch and Dinner Food Choices at
Selected Fast-Food Restaurants (continued)

FOOD ITEM	SERVING SIZE`	KCAL	CARBO-HYDRATE	PROTEIN	FAT	EXCHANGES
CARL'S JR. CONTINUED						
Lite potato	10 oz	290	83%	14%	3%	4 starch
Garden salad to go	4.8 oz	50	32%	14%	54%	1 vegetable
Chicken salad to go	12 oz	200	16%	48%	36%	1 vegetable, 3 lean meat
Reduced-calorie French dressing	1 oz	40	55%	0%	45%	1 fat
Salsa	1 oz	8	100%	—	—	—
KENTUCKY FRIED CHICKEN						
Side items that are low in fat and high in carbohydrate:						
Corn on cob	2.6 oz	90	71%	8%	20%	1 starch
Baked beans	3 oz	105	69%	23%	8%	1 starch
Mashed potatoes with gravy	3.5 oz	71	68%	7%	25%	1 starch

> ✔ **Note:** Despite different coatings, all KFC chicken is fried. Therefore, calories from fat range between 48% and 59% (even skin-free crispy).

TABLE A-2
Lower-Fat, High-Carbohydrate Lunch and Dinner Food Choices at Selected Fast-Food Restaurants (continued)

FOOD ITEM	SERVING SIZE	KCAL	CARBO-HYDRATE	PROTEIN	FAT	EXCHANGES
McDONALD'S						
Hamburger	3.6 oz	255	47%	21%	32%	2 starch, 1 medium fat meat, 1 fat
McLean Deluxe	7.7 oz	320	44%	28%	28%	2 starch, 3 lean meat
Chicken fajitas	2.9 oz	190	42%	20%	38%	1 starch, 1 lean meat, 1 fat
Cheese pizza	2.6 oz (1 slice)	178	54%	11%	35%	1½ starch, 1 medium fat meat
Chunky chicken salad	9 oz	150	19%	57%	24%	1 vegetable, 3 lean meat
Garden salad	6.6 oz	50	48%	16%	36%	1 vegetable
Lite vinaigrette	2 oz	48	67%	0%	33%	1 fat
DOMINO'S PIZZA						
Cheese pizza	2 slices of a large (5.5 oz)	376	60%	16%	24%	4 starch, 2 medium fat meat
Vegetable pizza	2 slices of a large (5.5 oz)	498	48%	18%	34%	4 starch, 3 medium fat meat, 1 fat
Ham pizza	2 slices of medium pizza (5.5 oz)	417	55%	22%	23%	4 starch, 2 medium fat meat

TABLE A-2
Lower-Fat, High-Carbohydrate Lunch and Dinner Food Choices at Selected Fast-Food Restaurants (continued)

FOOD ITEM	SERVING SIZE	KCAL	CARBO-HYDRATE	PROTEIN	FAT	EXCHANGES
PIZZA HUT PIZZA						
Thin crispy:* Veggie Lover's pizza	*2 slices of medium pizza*	*384*	*42%*	*20%*	*38%*	*2 starch, 3 medium fat meat*
Cheese pizza	*2 slices of medium pizza*	*446*	*34%*	*26%*	*40%*	*2 starch, 3 medium fat meat, 2 fat*

* Hand-tossed pizza has similar values; pan pizza is significantly higher in calories.

TACO BELL						
Bean burrito	*6.7 oz*	*359*	*60%*	*12%*	*28%*	*3½ starch, 1 medium fat meat, 1 fat*
Chicken burrito	*6 oz*	*334*	*46%*	*22%*	*32%*	*2½ starch, 2 medium fat meat*
Border lights*	*(have 50% less fat than comparable products)*					
Light taco salad with chips	*21 oz*	*680*	*48%*	*19%*	*33%*	*5 starch, 3½ lean meat*
Light soft taco	*3.25 oz*	*180*	*42%*	*33%*	*25%*	*1 starch, 1½ lean meat*

* Available at selected locations

TABLE A-2
Lower-Fat, High-Carbohydrate Lunch and Dinner Food Choices at Selected Fast-Food Restaurants (continued)

FOOD ITEM	SERVING SIZE	KCAL	CARBO-HYDRATE	PROTEIN	FAT	EXCHANGES
WENDY'S						
Grilled hamburger	4 oz	270	50%	20%	30%	2 starch, 1½ medium fat meat
Grilled chicken sandwich	6.25 oz	290	48%	30%	22%	2 starch, 1 vegetable, 2 lean meat
Baked potato	10 oz	300	92%	7%	0%	4 starch
Chili	8 oz (small)	190	44%	28%	28%	1½ starch, 2 lean meat
Grilled chicken salad	12 oz	200	18%	46%	36%	2 vegetable, 3 lean meat

At the salad bar, avoid higher-fat items such as:

Bacon bits
Cheese
Coleslaw
Chicken, seafood, tuna salad (with oil or mayonnaise)
Potato, pasta salad (with oil or mayonnaise)
Pepperoni
Luncheon meats, diced
Nuts

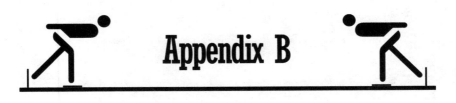

CALORIC EXPENDITURES

The following table lists approximate caloric expenditures per minute for various physical activities.

APPENDIX B: APPROXIMATE CALORIC EXPENDITURE PER MINUTE FOR VARIOUS PHYSICAL ACTIVITIES*

| Body weight in kilograms | 45 | 50 | 55 | 59 | 64 | 68 | 73 | 77 | 82 | 86 | 91 | 95 | 100 |
Body weight in pounds	100	110	120	130	140	150	160	170	180	190	200	210	220
SEDENTARY ACTIVITIES													
Lying quietly	.99	1.1	1.2	1.3	1.4	1.5	1.6	1.7	1.8	1.9	2.0	2.1	2.2
Sitting and writing	1.2	1.4	1.5	1.7	1.8	1.9	2.0	2.2	2.3	2.4	2.5	2.7	2.8
Standing with light work	2.7	3.0	3.3	3.5	3.8	4.1	4.4	4.6	4.9	5.2	5.4	5.7	6.0
PHYSICAL ACTIVITIES													
Archery	3.1	3.5	3.8	4.1	4.5	4.8	5.1	5.4	5.7	6.0	6.4	6.7	7.0
Badminton													
Recreational singles	3.6	4.0	4.4	4.7	5.1	5.4	5.8	6.2	6.6	6.9	7.3	7.6	8.0
Competitive	5.9	6.4	7.0	7.6	8.2	8.8	9.4	10.0	10.6	11.2	11.8	12.4	13.0
Baseball													
Player	3.1	3.4	3.8	4.1	4.4	4.7	5.0	5.3	5.6	5.9	6.3	6.6	6.9
Pitcher	3.9	4.3	4.7	5.1	5.5	5.9	6.3	6.7	7.1	7.4	7.9	8.2	8.6
Basketball													
Recreational	4.9	5.5	6.0	6.5	7.0	7.5	8.0	8.5	9.0	9.5	10.0	10.5	11.0
Vigorous competition	6.5	7.2	7.8	8.5	9.2	9.9	10.5	11.2	11.9	12.5	13.2	13.8	14.5
Bicycling, level (mph) (min / mile)													
5 12:00	1.9	2.1	2.3	2.5	2.7	2.9	3.1	3.3	3.5	3.7	3.9	4.1	4.3
10 6:00	4.2	4.6	5.1	5.5	5.9	6.4	6.8	7.2	7.6	8.1	8.5	8.9	9.4
15 4:00	7.3	8.0	8.7	9.5	10.0	10.9	11.6	12.4	13.1	13.8	14.5	15.3	16.0
20 3:00	10.7	11.7	12.8	13.9	14.9	16.0	17.1	18.1	19.2	20.3	21.3	22.4	23.5
Canoeing (mph) (min / mile)													
2.5 24	1.9	2.1	2.3	2.5	2.7	2.9	3.1	3.3	3.5	3.7	3.9	4.1	4.3
4.0 15	4.4	4.9	5.3	5.8	6.2	6.7	7.1	7.6	8.0	8.5	8.9	9.4	9.8
5.0 12	5.7	6.3	6.9	7.5	8.1	8.7	9.3	9.8	10.4	11.0	11.6	12.2	12.8

Adapted from Williams, M. H. *Nutrition for Fitness and Sport*, 3rd ed. Wm. C. Brown Publishers, 1992.

APPENDIX B: APPROXIMATE CALORIC EXPENDITURE PER MINUTE FOR VARIOUS PHYSICAL ACTIVITIES*(Continued)

| Body weight in kilograms | 45 | 50 | 55 | 59 | 64 | 68 | 73 | 77 | 82 | 86 | 91 | 95 | 100 |
Body weight in pounds	100	110	120	130	140	150	160	170	180	190	200	210	220
Dancing													
Moderately (waltz)	3.1	3.5	3.8	4.1	4.5	4.8	5.1	5.4	5.7	6.0	6.4	6.7	7.0
Active (square, disco)	4.5	5.0	5.4	5.9	6.3	6.8	7.3	7.7	8.2	8.6	9.1	9.5	10.0
Aerobic (vigorously)	6.0	6.7	7.3	7.9	8.5	9.1	9.7	10.3	10.9	11.5	12.1	12.7	13.3
Fencing													
Moderately	3.3	3.6	4.0	4.3	4.6	5.0	5.3	5.7	6.0	6.3	6.7	7.0	7.3
Vigorously	6.6	7.3	8.0	8.7	9.4	10.0	10.7	11.4	12.1	12.7	13.4	14.1	14.8
Football													
Moderate	3.3	3.6	4.0	4.3	4.6	5.0	5.3	5.7	6.0	6.3	6.7	7.0	7.3
Touch, vigorous	5.5	6.1	6.6	7.2	7.8	8.3	8.9	9.4	10.0	10.6	11.1	11.7	12.2
Golf													
Twosome (carry clubs)	3.6	4.0	4.4	4.7	5.1	5.4	5.8	6.2	6.6	6.9	7.3	7.6	8.0
Foursome (carry clubs)	2.7	3.0	3.3	3.5	3.8	4.1	4.4	4.6	4.9	5.2	5.4	5.7	6.0
Power-cart	1.9	2.1	2.3	2.5	2.7	2.9	3.1	3.3	3.5	3.7	3.9	4.1	4.3
Handball													
Moderate	6.5	7.2	7.8	8.5	9.2	9.9	10.5	11.2	11.9	12.5	13.2	13.8	14.5
Competitive	7.7	8.4	9.2	10.0	10.8	11.5	12.3	13.1	13.9	14.7	15.4	16.2	17.0
Hiking, pack (3 mph)	4.5	5.0	5.4	5.9	6.3	6.8	7.3	7.7	8.2	8.6	9.1	9.5	10.0
Hockey, field	5.0	6.7	7.3	7.9	8.5	9.1	9.7	10.3	10.9	11.5	12.1	12.7	13.3
Hockey, ice	6.6	7.3	8.0	8.7	9.4	10.0	10.7	11.4	12.1	12.7	13.4	14.1	14.8
Horseback riding													
Walk	1.9	2.1	2.3	2.5	2.7	2.9	3.1	3.3	3.5	3.7	3.9	4.1	4.3
Sitting to trot	2.7	3.0	3.3	3.5	3.8	4.1	4.4	4.6	4.9	5.2	5.4	5.7	6.0
Posting to trot	4.2	4.6	5.1	5.5	5.9	6.4	6.8	7.2	7.6	8.1	8.5	8.9	9.4
Gallop	5.7	6.3	6.9	7.5	8.1	8.7	9.3	9.8	10.4	11.0	11.6	12.2	12.8

APPENDIX B: APPROXIMATE CALORIC EXPENDITURE PER MINUTE FOR VARIOUS PHYSICAL ACTIVITIES* (Continued)

| Body weight in kilograms | 45 | 50 | 55 | 59 | 64 | 68 | 73 | 77 | 82 | 86 | 91 | 95 | 100 |
Body weight in pounds	100	110	120	130	140	150	160	170	180	190	200	210	220
Jogging (see Running)													
Judo	8.5	9.3	10.2	11.0	11.9	12.8	13.6	14.5	15.4	16.2	17.1	17.9	18.8
Karate	8.5	9.3	10.2	11.0	11.9	12.8	13.6	14.5	15.4	16.2	17.1	17.9	18.8
Mountain climbing	6.5	7.2	7.8	8.5	9.2	9.8	10.5	11.2	11.8	12.5	13.1	13.8	14.5
Paddle ball	5.7	6.3	6.9	7.5	8.1	8.7	9.3	9.8	10.4	11.0	11.6	12.2	12.8
Racketball	6.5	7.1	7.8	8.4	9.1	9.8	10.4	11.1	11.7	12.4	13.0	13.7	14.4
Roller skating (9 mph)	4.2	4.6	5.1	5.5	5.9	6.4	6.8	7.2	7.6	8.1	8.5	8.9	9.4
Running (steady state)													
(mph) (min / mile)													
5.0 12:00	6.0	6.6	7.3	7.9	8.5	9.1	9.7	10.3	10.9	11.6	12.2	12.8	13.4
5.5 10:55	6.7	7.3	8.0	8.7	9.4	10.0	10.7	11.4	12.1	12.8	13.4	14.1	14.8
6.0 10:00	7.2	8.0	8.7	9.5	10.2	10.9	11.7	12.4	13.1	13.8	14.6	15.4	16.1
7.0 8:35	8.5	9.3	10.2	11.0	11.9	12.8	13.6	14.5	15.4	16.2	17.1	17.9	18.8
8.0 7:30	9.7	10.7	11.6	12.6	13.6	14.6	15.6	16.6	17.6	18.5	19.5	20.5	21.5
9.0 6:40	10.8	11.9	12.9	14.0	15.1	16.2	17.3	18.4	19.5	20.6	21.7	22.8	23.9
10.0 6:00	12.1	13.3	14.5	15.7	17.0	18.2	19.4	20.7	21.9	23.1	24.2	25.4	26.7
11.0 5:28	13.3	14.6	16.0	17.3	18.7	20.0	21.4	22.7	24.1	25.4	26.8	28.1	29.5
12.0 5:00	14.5	16.0	17.4	18.9	20.4	21.9	23.3	24.8	26.3	27.8	29.2	30.7	32.2
Skating, ice (9 mph)	4.2	4.6	5.1	5.5	5.9	6.4	6.8	7.2	7.6	8.1	8.5	8.9	9.4
Skiing, cross country													
(mph) (min / mile)													
2.5 24:00	5.0	5.5	6.0	6.5	7.0	7.5	8.0	8.5	9.0	9.5	10.0	10.6	11.1
4.0 15:00	6.5	7.2	7.8	8.5	9.2	9.9	10.5	11.2	11.9	12.5	13.2	13.8	14.5
5.0 12:00	7.7	8.4	9.2	10.0	10.8	11.5	12.3	13.1	13.9	14.7	15.4	16.2	17.0
Skiing, downhill	6.5	7.2	7.8	8.5	9.2	9.9	10.5	11.2	11.9	12.5	13.2	13.8	14.5

APPENDIX B: APPROXIMATE CALORIC EXPENDITURE PER MINUTE FOR VARIOUS PHYSICAL ACTIVITIES* (Continued)

| Body weight in kilograms | 45 | 50 | 55 | 59 | 64 | 68 | 73 | 77 | 82 | 86 | 91 | 95 | 100 |
Body weight in pounds	100	110	120	130	140	150	160	170	180	190	200	210	220
Soccer	5.9	6.6	7.2	7.8	8.4	9.0	9.6	10.2	10.8	11.4	12.0	12.6	13.2
Squash													
Normal	6.7	7.3	8.0	8.7	9.5	10.1	10.8	11.5	12.2	12.9	13.5	14.2	14.9
Competition	7.7	8.4	9.2	10.0	10.8	11.5	12.3	13.1	13.9	14.7	15.4	16.2	17.0
Swimming (yards/mi)													
Backstroke													
25	2.5	2.8	3.0	3.3	3.5	3.8	4.0	4.3	4.5	4.8	5.1	5.3	5.6
30	3.5	3.9	4.2	4.6	4.9	5.3	5.6	6.0	6.4	6.7	7.1	7.4	7.8
35	4.5	5.0	5.4	5.9	6.3	6.8	7.3	7.7	8.2	8.6	9.1	9.5	10.0
40	5.5	6.1	6.6	7.2	7.8	8.3	8.9	9.4	10.0	10.6	11.1	11.7	12.2
Breaststroke													
20	3.1	3.5	3.8	4.1	4.5	4.8	5.1	5.4	5.7	6.0	6.4	6.7	7.0
30	4.7	5.2	5.7	6.2	6.7	7.1	7.6	8.1	8.6	9.1	9.5	10.0	10.5
40	6.3	7.0	7.6	8.3	8.9	9.6	10.2	10.9	11.5	12.2	12.8	13.5	14.1
Front crawl													
20	3.1	3.5	3.8	4.1	4.5	4.8	5.1	5.4	5.7	6.0	6.4	6.7	7.0
25	4.0	4.4	4.8	5.2	5.6	6.0	6.4	6.8	7.2	7.6	8.0	8.4	8.8
35	4.8	5.4	5.9	6.4	6.8	7.3	7.8	8.3	8.8	9.2	9.7	10.2	10.7
45	5.7	6.3	6.9	7.5	8.1	8.7	9.3	9.8	10.4	11.0	11.6	12.2	12.8
50	7.0	7.7	8.5	9.2	9.9	10.6	11.3	12.0	12.8	13.5	14.2	14.9	15.6
Table tennis	3.4	3.8	4.1	4.5	4.8	5.2	5.5	5.9	6.3	6.6	7.0	7.3	7.7
Tennis													
Singles (recreational)	5.0	5.5	6.0	6.5	7.0	7.5	8.0	8.5	9.0	9.5	10.0	10.6	11.1
Competition	6.4	7.1	7.7	8.4	9.1	9.8	10.4	11.1	11.8	12.4	13.1	13.7	14.4

APPENDIX B: APPROXIMATE CALORIC EXPENDITURE PER MINUTE FOR VARIOUS PHYSICAL ACTIVITIES*(Continued)

| Body weight in kilograms | 45 | 50 | 55 | 59 | 64 | 68 | 73 | 77 | 82 | 86 | 91 | 95 | 100 |
Body weight in pounds	100	110	120	130	140	150	160	170	180	190	200	210	220
Volleyball													
Moderate recreational	2.9	3.2	3.5	3.8	4.1	4.4	4.7	5.0	5.3	5.6	5.9	6.1	6.4
Vigorous, competition	6.5	7.1	7.8	8.4	9.1	9.8	10.4	11.1	11.7	12.4	13.0	13.7	14.4
Walking													
(mph) (min / mile)													
2.0 30:00	2.1	2.3	2.5	2.8	3.0	3.2	3.4	3.6	3.9	4.1	4.3	4.5	4.7
3.0 20:00	2.7	3.0	3.3	3.5	3.8	4.1	4.4	4.6	4.9	5.2	5.4	5.7	6.0
3.5 17.10	3.3	3.7	4.0	4.4	4.7	5.1	5.4	5.8	6.2	6.5	6.9	7.2	7.6
4.0 15:00	4.2	4.6	5.1	5.5	5.9	6.4	6.8	7.2	7.6	8.1	8.5	8.9	9.4
4.5 13.20	4.7	5.2	5.7	6.2	6.7	7.1	7.6	8.1	8.6	9.1	9.5	10.0	10.5
5.0 12:00	5.4	6.0	6.5	7.1	7.7	8.2	8.7	9.2	9.8	10.4	10.9	11.5	12.0
5.4 11:10	6.2	6.9	7.5	8.2	8.8	9.5	10.1	10.3	11.4	12.1	12.7	13.4	14.0
5.8 10:20	7.7	8.4	9.2	10.0	10.8	11.5	12.3	13.1	13.9	14.7	15.4	16.2	17.0
Water skiing	5.0	5.5	6.0	6.5	7.0	7.5	8.0	8.5	9.0	9.5	10.0	10.6	11.1
Weight training	5.2	5.7	6.2	6.8	7.3	7.8	8.3	8.9	9.4	9.9	10.5	11.0	11.5
Wrestling	8.5	9.3	10.2	11.0	11.9	12.8	13.6	14.5	15.4	16.2	17.1	17.9	18.8

✔ **Note:** The energy cost, in calories, will vary for different physical activities in a given individual depending on several factors. For example, the caloric cost of bicycling will vary depending on the type of bicycle, going uphill or downhill, and wind resistance. Walking with hand weights or ankle weights will increase energy output. Thus, the values expressed here are approximations and may be increased or decreased depending upon factors that influence energy cost.

ABOUT THE AUTHORS

Ellen Coleman, RD, MA, MPH, is an exercise physiologist and registered dietitian. She is a columnist for *Sports Medicine Digest* and Nutrition Consultant for the S.P.O.R.T. Clinic in Riverside, California. She received the 1994 Achievement Award from the SCAN Practice Group of the American Dietetic Association. Ellen has completed the Ironman Triathlon in Hawaii twice and numerous marathons and 200-mile bicycle races. She is the author of *Eating for Endurance*. Ellen counsels endurance athletes and professional athletes.

Suzanne Nelson Steen, DSc, RD, is Assistant Professor at Immaculata College, Department of Nutrition Education, Immaculata, Pennsylvania. She is co-author of *Play Hard Eat Right—A Parents' Guide to Sports Nutrition for Children,* and co-editor of *Sports Nutrition for the 90's.* She has published numerous scientific articles and book chapters. Suzanne counsels child athletes, collegiate athletes, and olympic athletes.

INDEX